Veterinary Dentistry for the Nurse and Technician

For Butterworth Heinemann:

Commissioning Editor: Mary Seager
Development Editor: Rita Demetriou-Swanwick
Project Manager: Joannah Duncan
Designer: Andy Chapman
Illustration Manager: Bruce Hogarth

Veterinary Dentistry for the Nurse and Technician

Cecilia Gorrel BSc MA VetMB DDS HonFAVD DiplEVDC MRCVS

Veterinary Dentistry and Oral Surgery Referrals,
Veterinary Oral Health Consultancy, Pilley, UK

Sue Derbyshire VN PHC

Veterinary Dentistry and Oral Surgery Referrals,
Pilley, UK

ELSEVIER
BUTTERWORTH
HEINEMANN

Edinburgh London New York Oxford Philadelphia St Louis Sydney Toronto 2005

ELSEVIER
BUTTERWORTH
HEINEMANN

First published 2005

ISBN 0 7506 5286 1

British Library Cataloguing in Publication Data
A catalogue record for this book is available from the British Library

Library of Congress Cataloging in Publication Data
A catalog record for this book is available from the Library of Congress

Knowledge and best practice in this field are constantly changing. As new research and experience broaden our knowledge, changes in practice, treatment and drug therapy may become necessary or appropriate. Readers are advised to check the most current information provided (i) on procedures featured or (ii) by the manufacturer of each product to be administered, to verify the recommended dose or formula, the method and duration of administration, and contraindications. It is the responsibility of the practitioner, relying on their own experience and knowledge of the patient, to make diagnoses, to determine dosages and the best treatment for each individual patient, and to take all appropriate safety precautions. To the fullest extent of the law, neither the publisher nor the authors assume any liability for any injury and/or damage.

The Publisher

Contents

Preface

This book was written for the veterinary nurse and technician in a small animal practice. The nurse and technician are essential members of an effective oral care team, yet oral health and disease is often not covered in nursing and technician training programmes. (*Note*: in the US the term veterinary technician is used rather than veterinary nurse.)

The veterinarian is responsible for diagnosis and treatment of oral diseases. The trained veterinary nurse and technician assist the veterinarian in these duties but also perform dental hygiene instruction and treatment as requested by the veterinarian. In other words the trained nurse and technician take on the role of 'dental nurse' and 'dental hygienist'. The nurse and technician can only perform these duties if requested to do so by the veterinarian and then only under direct supervision of the veterinarian. Moreover, the veterinarian is accountable for the adequacy of any procedures performed by the nurse and technician.

The trained nurse and technician should be able to carry out the following procedures:

- Perform an oral examination
- Record findings on a dental chart
- Take dental radiographs
- Perform routine periodontal therapy
- Perform oral/dental hygiene instruction

In addition, they are responsible for the care and maintenance of equipment and instrumentation.

We hope that all the information required to perform these duties is covered in this book.

Cecilia Gorrel and Sue Derbyshire
Pilley 2005

Acknowledgements

This book would not have been written without the assistance of Graeme Blackwood. Thank you for your emotional support and practical help. We also thank our proofreaders Katarina Gorrel and Amy Blackwood.

Together with Leen Verhaert, we wish to thank Professors Lauwers and Simons of the Morphology department, Faculty of Veterinary Medicine, Ghent University, for allowing us to take photographs of the skulls in the Department Museum.

1

The role of the veterinary nurse and technician

In human dentistry the primary team that supplies oral care consists of the dentist (general dental practitioner), the dental nurse, the dental hygienist and the dental technician. Each of these individuals has a clearly defined role. Namely, the dentist is responsible for oral diagnosis and treatment; the dental nurse assists the dentist in these duties; the dental hygienist performs dental hygiene instruction and treatment as requested by the dentist; and the dental technician manufactures appliances (crowns, inlays, bridges, prostheses) as requested by the dentist. In addition to this primary care team, there are specialists in the various dental disciplines (periodontics, orthodontics, endodontics, oral surgery, prosthodontics, etc.). The specialists provide treatment that is outside the scope of the general dental practitioner.

The veterinary oral care team is not as easy to define. Despite the fact that oral conditions are common in domestic pets, the education in veterinary dentistry and oral surgery is not a big part of the undergraduate veterinary curriculum. Consequently, many veterinarians are not comfortable in diagnosing oral conditions or in performing dental and oral surgery procedures. Moreover, dentistry is often not considered 'important' and is often delegated to nurses or technicians who have even less knowledge of the discipline. (*Note*: in the US the term veterinary technician is used rather than veterinary nurse.) In fact, oral health and disease is often not covered at all in the nursing and technician training programmes. This is an unfortunate situation and does not benefit the oral health and general welfare of our domestic pets. There is today an urgent need to provide education in dentistry and oral surgery for veterinarians as well as for nurses and technicians. Moreover, the role of the veterinary nurse and technician in the oral care team needs to be clearly defined.

In proposing the role of the veterinary nurse and technician in the field of veterinary dentistry and oral surgery, the legal situation must be considered. The legislation varies throughout the world. In the following, the legal situation in the UK will be detailed.

THE VETERINARY SURGEONS ACT

Under the Veterinary Surgeons Act 1966, the general rule is that only a veterinary surgeon may practise veterinary surgery. Veterinary surgery, as defined in the Act, 'means the art and science of veterinary surgery and medicine and, without prejudice to the generality of the foregoing, shall be taken to include:

(a) the diagnosis of disease in, and injuries to, animals including tests performed on animals for diagnostic purposes;
(b) the giving of advice based upon such diagnosis;

(c) the medical or surgical treatment of animals; and
(d) the performance of surgical operations on animals.'

Veterinary nurses may give first aid and look after animals in ways that do not involve acts of veterinary surgery. In addition, veterinary nurses may do the things specified in paragraphs 6 (applies to listed veterinary nurses) and 7 (applies to student veterinary nurses) of Schedule 3 to the Veterinary Surgeons Act 1966, as amended by the Veterinary Surgeons Act 1966 (Schedule 3 Amendment) Order 2002, SI 2002/1479, with effect from 10 June 2002. See Appendix 1 for full text.

THE VETERINARY ORAL CARE TEAM

In our view, veterinary oral care should be structured similarly to human oral care. Namely, the veterinarian is responsible for diagnosis and treatment; the veterinary nurse and technician assist the veterinarian in these duties, but also perform dental hygiene instruction and treatment as requested by the veterinarian. In other words, the veterinary nurse and technician take on the duties of 'dental nurse' as well as 'dental hygienist'. The nurse and technician can only perform these duties if specifically requested to do so by the veterinarian and then only under the direct supervision of the veterinarian. Moreover, the veterinarian is accountable for the adequacy of any procedures performed by the veterinary nurse and technician. In other words, the veterinarian is ultimately responsible.

In addition to the veterinarian in general practice, there are now veterinarians who are specialists in dentistry (Diplomates of the European Veterinary Dental College or of the American Veterinary Dental College). They provide treatment that is outside the scope of the general dental practitioner, e.g. complicated extractions and other surgical procedures, endodontics, prosthodontics, etc.

The veterinary nurse and technician are essential members of an effective oral care team. The trained veterinary nurse and technician should be able to carry out the following procedures:

- Perform an oral examination
- Record findings on a dental chart
- Take dental radiographs
- Perform routine periodontal therapy
- Perform oral/dental hygiene instruction

ORAL EXAMINATION AND RECORDING

Legally, the veterinary nurse cannot make a diagnosis. So, while examination of the oral cavity and recording of findings can be performed by the trained nurse and technician, these findings need to be verified by the veterinarian, who then makes the diagnosis and draws up the treatment plan.

RADIOGRAPHY

Similarly, while a nurse or technician can take radiographs, the interpretation of the films is the duty of the veterinarian. It is time effective for the nurse or technician to take the radiographs. It is recommended.

PERIODONTAL THERAPY

Professional periodontal therapy includes:

1. Supra- and subgingival scaling
2. Crown polishing
3. Root planing
4. Extraction
5. Periodontal surgery

The trained veterinary nurse and technician should be able to perform supra- and subgingival scaling, crown polishing and root planing at the request of, and under the supervision of, the veterinarian. The adequacy of the procedures needs to be checked by the veterinarian, who has the ultimate legal responsibility.

Extraction and periodontal surgery are the remit of the veterinarian. While a trained veterinary nurse and technician may legally (varies from country to country) be allowed to perform minor surgery at the request of the veterinarian, neither tooth extraction nor periodontal surgery can be considered as minor surgery. Tooth extraction is a commonly required procedure in veterinary dentistry. It is associated with a high risk of complications, many of which are iatrogenic in origin. In human dentistry, the general dental practitioner does perform simple extractions, but complicated extractions are often referred to a specialist in oral surgery. In people, periodontal surgery is generally the remit of a specialist in periodontology. Similarly in veterinary dentistry, a veterinarian (either the general practitioner or a specialist) should perform tooth extraction. The specialist in veterinary dentistry should manage patients requiring periodontal surgery.

The veterinary nurse and technician need to have knowledge of the different extraction techniques, as they are often required to assist the veterinarian in performing these procedures. Extraction techniques are detailed in Chapter 11. Simple extractions do not usually require assistance, but complicated extractions usually do. In fact, assistance greatly reduces trauma to the patient and speeds up the surgical procedure. It is strongly recommended.

ORAL/DENTAL HYGIENE INSTRUCTION

The trained veterinary nurse and technician have a crucial role to play in providing oral/dental hygiene instruction to pet owners. Preventive dentistry is detailed in Chapter 10. It is strongly recommended that the trained veterinary nurse and technician take on the responsibility of educating and training pet owners to perform optimal home care.

Every dog and cat requires daily home care. The regimen needs to be adapted to the individual needs of the animal. The adequacy of the home care provided by the owner needs to be assessed at regular intervals. It is recommended that owners of puppies and kittens receive dental hygiene education and instruction at the time of initial vaccination. The adequacy of the home care is then assessed 3–6 months later and an individual recall schedule is established. The trained veterinary nurse and technician should hold the appointments and run the clinics required for educating clients and for instructing and assessing home care.

Summary

- An effective primary oral care team consists of a trained veterinarian and trained nurses and technicians
- Trained veterinary nurses and technicians are essential members of an oral care team, taking on the duties of 'dental nurse' as well as 'dental hygienist'
- The veterinarian is responsible for diagnosis and treatment
- The nurse and technician assist the veterinarian in these duties and can also perform dental hygiene treatment and instruction as requested by the veterinarian
- Such procedures should be performed under the direct supervision of the veterinary surgeon
- The veterinarian is accountable for the adequacy of any procedures performed by veterinary nurses and technicians

2

Equipment and instrumentation

This chapter deals with important general considerations relating to the good practice of dentistry and oral surgery. It also details equipment and instrumentation requirements, as well as their care and maintenance. The additional requirements for lagomorphs and rodent dentistry are detailed in Chapter 12. Radiography is mandatory; equipment and techniques are covered in Chapter 7.

GENERAL CONSIDERATIONS

Since many dental procedures result in the creation of a bacterial aerosol, a separate room should be designated for oral and dental procedures. The room must have adequate light and ventilation. A dental light is mandatory.

Ergonomic considerations are of paramount importance in the layout of the dental operatory. All equipment and instruments should be within easy reach of the operator. Posture is important! Ideally, the operator should be seated.

It is essential to *protect operator and staff.* The operator and assistant(s) should wear facemasks and appropriate eye wear (spectacles or a face shield) to protect them from bacterial aerosol and debris. The oral cavity is never a sterile site, so the use of surgical gloves is recommended. If the operator works in a dirty environment without gloves, skin wounds are likely to get infected.

Important *patient considerations* are as follows:

- General anaesthesia with endotracheal intubation is essential. This prevents inhalation of aerosolised bacteria, debris and asphyxiation on irrigation and cooling fluids
- A pharyngeal pack is also recommended during oral and dental treatment. Remember to remove the pharyngeal pack prior to extubation! Chapter 3 covers anaesthesia and analgesia for the patient undergoing oral and dental surgery
- The animal should be positioned on a surface that will allow drainage to prevent it becoming wet and hypothermic. This can be achieved by the use of a 'tub-tank' or by placing the animal's head on a towel or disposable 'nappy'. Most animals benefit from a heating pad

Some important *equipment and instrumentation considerations* are as follows:

- Clean, sterilised instruments should be available for each patient. Ideally, several pre-packed kits containing the required instruments for the different procedures (e.g. examination, periodontal therapy, extraction), should be available
- Power equipment requires regular maintenance (daily, weekly) in the practice and regular servicing by the supplier. Draw up checklists for these chores. Check maintenance and servicing requirements with the supplier

EQUIPMENT AND INSTRUMENTATION FOR ORAL AND DENTAL EXAMINATION

The details of how to perform oral examination and recording are covered in Chapter 6. The following will outline equipment and instrumentation requirements. Personal preferences have been inserted as a guide, where appropriate.

Periodontal probe

The periodontal probe is a narrow rounded or flat, blunt-ended, graduated instrument. Due to its blunt end, it can be inserted into the gingival sulcus without causing trauma (Fig. 2.1). The periodontal probe is used to:

- Measure periodontal probing depth
- Determine degree of gingival inflammation
- Evaluate furcation lesions
- Evaluate extent of tooth mobility

A rounded narrow probe (e.g. No. 14 Williams B) is our preferred choice, as it is easier to enter the gingival sulcus without causing damage. This is especially true in cats, where the flat probe is impossible to use.

Dental explorer

The dental explorer or probe, a sharp-ended instrument, is used to:

- Determine the presence of caries
- Explore other enamel and dentine defects, e.g. fracture, odontoclastic resorptive lesions

The explorer is also useful for tactile examination of the subgingival tooth surfaces. Subgingival calculus and odontoclastic resorptive lesions may be identified in this way.

Dental explorers are either straight or curved (Fig. 2.2). They are also either single-ended or double-ended, usually combined with a periodontal probe, i.e. one end is an explorer and the other end is a periodontal probe. We use Explorer probe No. 6, a single-ended straight explorer.

Dental mirror

A dental mirror (Fig. 2.3) is a vital, but traditionally rarely used, tool in veterinary dentistry. It allows the operator to visualise palatal/lingual surfaces while maintaining posture. The dental mirror can also be used to reflect light onto areas

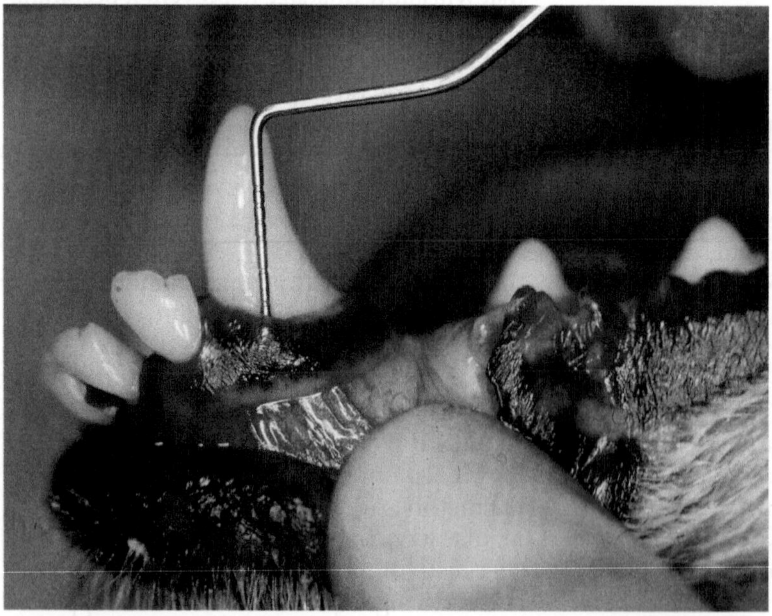

Fig. 2.1 The periodontal probe. The periodontal probe is a blunt-ended, graduated instrument, which can be inserted into the gingival sulcus without causing trauma.

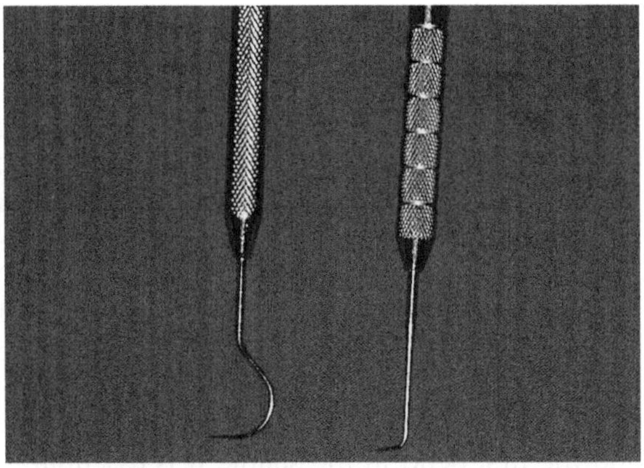

Fig. 2.2 The dental explorer. The dental explorer is either straight or curved (shepherd's hook). The use of double-ended explorers/probes is not recommended, due to the risk of inadvertent damage to the animal with the end not being used in the oral cavity.

of interest and to retract and protect soft tissue. Orientation may cause confusion and the use of a dental mirror requires practice. The time taken to learn how to use a dental mirror is a worthwhile investment. The mirror can be wiped across the buccal mucous membranes before use to prevent condensation occurring. Dental mirrors are available in several sizes. A small (paediatric size) mirror for cats and small dogs and a larger one for medium to large dogs should be available.

Dental record sheets

Recording and dental record sheets are covered in Chapter 6. A complete dental record is required for diagnostic and therapeutic purposes, as well as for medicolegal reasons.

EQUIPMENT AND INSTRUMENTATION FOR PERIODONTAL THERAPY

Periodontal therapy is detailed in Chapter 8.

Scaling

Scaling describes the procedure whereby dental deposits (plaque, but mainly calculus) are removed from the supra- and subgingival surfaces of the teeth. Scaling may be performed using a combination of mechanical and hand instruments. The use of mechanical (powered scalers) requires less treatment time than hand instruments. Moreover, mechanical instrumentation is less fatiguing to the operator than hand instrumentation. However, mechanical scalers cannot replace hand scaling. If only powered scalers have been used, post-treatment examination using compressed air to retract tissues and dry calculus demonstrates residual deposits. Hand instruments allow the operator to detect the texture and character of calculus deposits. Sometimes mechanical scalers will plane over the surface of a calculus rather than dislodge it. The sharpened blade of a hand instrument is more likely to break the calculus away from the tooth surface. Hand instruments should be used to remove large, bulky supragingival deposits before going on to powered scalers. Also, hand instruments are required to remove subgingival dental deposits.

Hand scaling instruments

Scalers and curettes (Fig. 2.4) are used to remove dental deposits from the tooth surfaces. Each has a handle, a shank and a working end (tip) (Fig. 2.5).

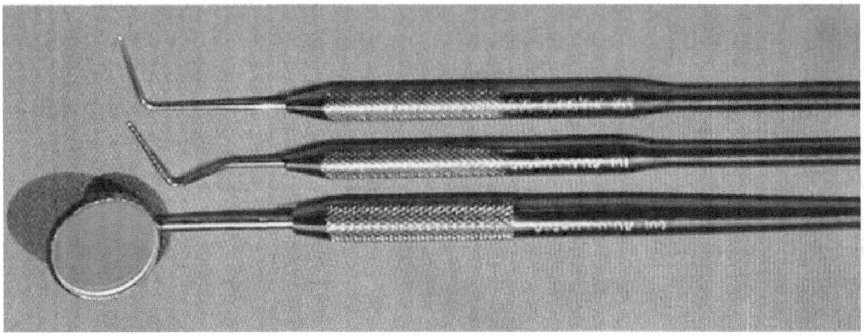

Fig. 2.3 The dental mirror. A dental mirror is a vital tool. It allows the operator to visualise palatal/lingual surfaces while maintaining posture, reflect light onto areas of interest, and retract and protect soft tissue. Also shown are a periodontal probe and a straight dental explorer. (Slide courtesy of Big-O, Veterinary Dental Supplies Company.)

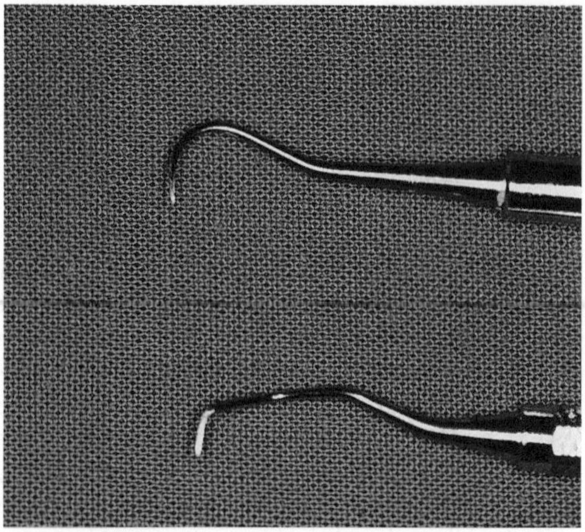

Fig. 2.4 Scaler and curette. The scaler (top) can only be used to remove supragingival dental deposits. The curette (bottom) is used to remove subgingival deposits and restore the root surface to smoothness. It can also be used to remove supragingival dental deposits.

They require frequent sharpening to maintain their cutting edges. Instrument sharpening is covered in the 'Sharpening' section later in this chapter.

Instrument (scaler and curette) handles are available in a variety of shapes and styles. Weight, diameter and surface texture of handles are factors that need to be considered when selecting hand instruments. Round, hollow handles are recommended because they are lighter in weight, which increases tactile sense, and minimises hand fatigue. A larger diameter handle is advisable for ergonomic comfort. A handle with a smooth surface must be grasped more firmly to maintain control over the working end, leading to hand fatigue. Textured handles (ribbed, diamond-textured or knurled) allow the operator to maintain control over the instrument more comfortably. They also maximise sensory feedback.

The part of the instrument that extends from the working end to the handle is called the functional shank. Functional shanks may be angled, curved or straight. They also vary in length (short, moderate, long) and flexibility. Straight shank instruments are commonly used on the accessible anterior teeth. Posterior teeth need angled shanks for better adaptation of the working end to the tooth surfaces. Instruments with short functional shanks can be used on anterior teeth, while moderate to long shanks are needed to reach posterior teeth and to access periodontal pockets. Instruments with rigid shanks are used to remove heavy calculus deposits. Instruments with more flexible shanks (e.g. Gracey curettes) are used for removal of fine, light calculus and give better tactile sensation (feedback). The terminal shank is the smaller portion of the functional shank. It extends between the working end and the first bend in the shank. It is essential to locate the terminal shank on an instrument when you are trying to identify the working end and sharpen its cutting edges.

The working end refers to that part of the instrument that is used to carry out the function of the instrument. Working ends can be made of stainless steel or of carbide steel. The working end of a sharpened instrument is called the blade. Carbide blades may hold their cutting edge(s) longer but tend to corrode easily if not cared for properly. The blade is made up of the following components:

- Face
- Lateral surfaces
- Back
- Cutting edge(s)

The cutting edge is the line where the face and a lateral surface meet to form a sharp cutting edge. A blade designed with a pointed tip is called a *scaler*. A blade that ends with a rounded toe is classified as a *curette*. Figure 2.5 demonstrates the differences between a scaler and a curette.

Scalers are used for the supragingival removal of calculus. As already mentioned, a scaler has a sharp, pointed tip and should thus only be used supragingivally. If a scaler is used subgingivally, the pointed tip will lacerate the gingival margin. A scaler should generally be pulled away from the gingiva towards the tip of the crown (occlusal surface).

Scalers come in a variety of shapes. The most common is the sickle scaler, which can be either curved or straight. A straight sickle scaler is also

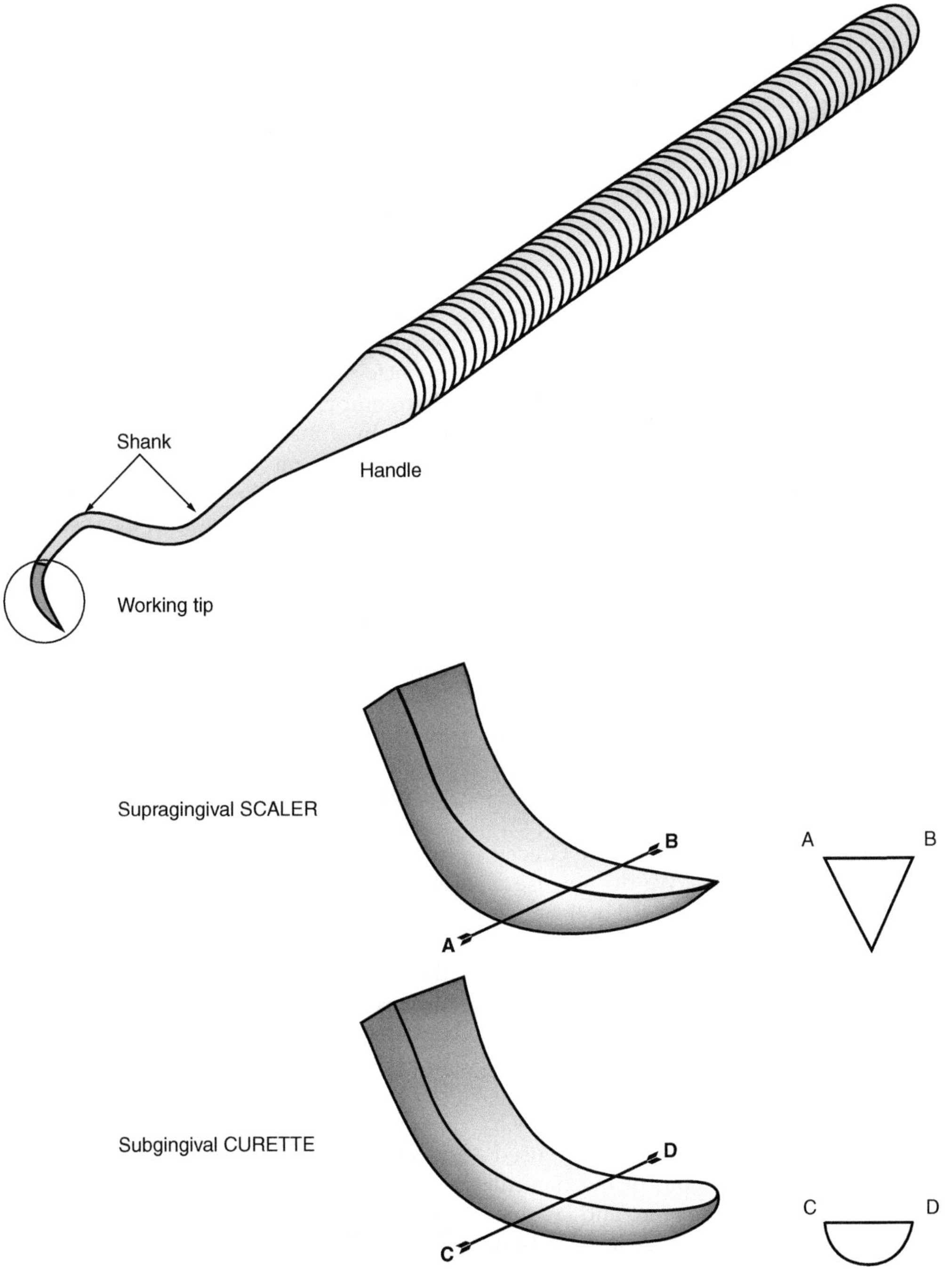

Fig. 2.5 Scaler and curette design. Each has a handle, a shank and a working tip. The working tip of a scaler is more robust than a curette. Curettes are less bulky, with rounded back and tip, for use in gingival pockets. Both hand scalers and curettes require frequent sharpening to maintain their cutting edges.

known as a jacquette scaler. A sickle scaler has the following characteristics:

1. The face of the blade is perpendicular to the terminal shank
2. The blade has two cutting edges
3. The face of the blade has a sharp point or tip
4. In cross-section, the blade is triangular in shape

Other types of scalers are hoes, chisels and files. Chisels and files are rarely used. The hoe, however, is a good instrument for removing large accessible amounts of calculus. The blade of a hoe has a 99 to 100° angle to the shank; the shape is reminiscent of a garden hoe. The width of the blade is applied at the gingival edge of the deposit, and a pull stroke is applied towards the occlusal surface.

Curettes are used for the subgingival removal of dental deposits and for root planing. They can also be used supragingivally. There are basically two types of curettes, namely universal and area specific, e.g. Gracey. The working end of a curette is more slender than that of a scaler and the back and tip are rounded to minimise gingival trauma. The cutting edges curve from the terminal shank to the toe.

A selection of curettes is required for periodontal therapy. Our preferences are the Gracey 7/8 and the Columbia 13/14. We do not use a separate scaler as curettes can be used both above and below the gingiva, whereas scalers are limited to supragingival use.

Mechanical scaling instruments

Mechanical or powered scalers enable fast and easy removal of calculus. However, they have a great potential for iatrogenic damage if used incorrectly. There are three types of mechanical scalers, namely sonic, ultrasonic and rotary. Gross supragingival calculus deposits are best removed with hand instruments (scaler, curette) prior to using mechanical scaling equipment.

Sonic scalers are driven by compressed air, so they require a compressed air driven dental unit (see 'Compressed air driven unit' section later in this chapter) for operation. The tip oscillates at a sonic frequency and is efficient at removing dental calculus. Sonic scalers are generally less effective than ultrasonic scalers, but generate less heat and are thus less likely to cause iatrogenic injuries and are, therefore, safer to use. Depending upon the design of the tip of the scaler, these instruments may be used for supra- and subgingival scaling. An insert with a thin, pointed tip (sometimes called a perio, sickle or universal insert) is our recommendation.

Ultrasonic scalers are commonly used in veterinary practice. The tip oscillates at ultrasonic frequencies. They are driven by a micromotor rather than compressed air. The tip vibration is generated either by a magnetostrictive mechanism, or by a piezoelectric mechanism in the handpiece. The ultrasonic oscillation of the tip causes cavitation of the coolant, which aids in the disruption of the calculus on the tooth surface. Ultrasonic scalers are generally designed for supragingival use, but tips designed for subgingival scaling are available. A thin, pointed insert is recommended for supragingival use. Inserts specifically designed for subgingival use are recommended for subgingival scaling. We have no real preference between sonic or ultrasonic scalers and use both.

Rotary scalers are best avoided, but are included here for completeness. In this system, roto pro burs are inserted in the high-speed handpiece of a compressed air driven unit. They are so-called 'non-cutting' burs, which when applied to calculus cause it to disintegrate while the coolant flushes the debris away. In humans, the use of these burs to scale teeth is associated with significant postoperative pain. They are thus no longer used for scaling. In addition to postoperative pain, roto pro burs can cause extensive damage to tooth enamel. Their use in veterinary dentistry is not recommended.

Calculus forceps

Calculus forceps have been designed to remove heavy calculus deposits. They must not be used to extract teeth. Calculus forceps have a long, straight beak and a shorter, curved beak. The long beak is placed on the occlusal surface of the tooth and the short beak is engaged below the calculus (but above the gingival margin) and the forceps are gently closed, thus crushing the calculus and scraping it off. It is essential to use these forceps with extreme care and in the described manner, as inappropriate use will result in fractured teeth. We generally do not use calculus forceps. Instead, gross calculus is removed using extraction forceps, which are gently closed around the tooth over the calculus while taking care not to damage the gingival margin.

Polishing

Polishing removes plaque and restores the scaled tooth surfaces to smoothness, which is less plaque retentive. Scaled teeth must be polished. It is often suggested that teeth may be 'polished' by hand using a toothbrush and prophy paste. This method is inefficient and, therefore, not recommended. Efficient polishing can be performed either using prophy paste in a prophy cup or in a brush in a slow-speed contra-angle handpiece, or by means of particle blasting (air polishing).

Prophy paste in a cup or brush in a slow-speed contra-angle handpiece

The speed of rotation of the cup or brush can be regulated. To minimise the amount of heat generated, the prophy cup or brush should not rotate faster than 1000 rpm (revolutions per minute). We prefer to use a soft cup rather than a brush. By exerting gentle pressure against the tooth, the soft cup can be made to flare out and thus polish tooth surfaces just below the gingival margin. Each patient should receive a new polishing cup.

Air polishing (particle blasting)

This technique, based on the sandblasting principle, is used to polish the supragingival parts of the teeth. The particles used (e.g. bicarbonate of soda) will polish the tooth surface without causing damage to the enamel, if used properly. It is essential to protect the soft tissues (gingivae and oral mucosa) during air polishing. A simple way of protecting the soft tissues is to cover them with a piece of gauze.

Prophy paste

Prophy paste is available in bulk containers and individual patient tubs. The latter are inexpensive and should be used to prevent contamination and iatrogenic transmission of pathogens.

EQUIPMENT AND INSTRUMENTATION FOR TOOTH EXTRACTION

The techniques for tooth extraction are detailed in Chapter 11.

Hand instruments

Hand instruments required for tooth extraction include a selection of luxators and elevators, periosteal elevators, possibly extraction forceps and a small surgical kit (scalpel blade, forceps, suturing instruments and suturing material).

Luxators and elevators

Luxators and elevators are used to cut or break down the periodontal ligament, which holds the tooth in the alveolus. A selection of dental luxators and elevators of varying sizes is required (Fig. 2.6), so that an appropriate range for each size of root can be selected. Luxators have a very thin working end and are used to cut the periodontal ligament, but should not be used for leverage or they may break. Elevators have thicker working ends. They are used to break down the periodontal ligament with a combination of apical pressure and leverage. An extraction can be started with a luxator and completed with an elevator. A very small (2 mm) luxator, or a root tip elevator, will assist removal of fractured root tips and should be available for all extractions – just in case!

Periosteal elevator

A periosteal elevator (Fig. 2.7) is required for open (surgical) extractions to expose the alveolar bone by raising a mucoperiosteal flap. However, even if a closed (non-surgical) extraction technique has been used, the gingiva may be sutured over the extraction socket. In this situation, a periosteal elevator is invaluable to free sufficient gingiva to allow tension-free closure.

Extraction forceps

Although forceps (Fig. 2.8) can be used to aid ligament breakdown by rotational force on the tooth, it is easy to snap the crown off by using excessive force. There is some truth in the saying that the only extraction forceps required are your fingers. If the tooth cannot be lifted out with your fingers, then the periodontal ligament has not been adequately broken down. In short, dental forceps are not essential, but if they are to be used a selection of sizes, to fit the root anatomy of the tooth being extracted, is required. We do not use extraction forceps for tooth extraction. Instead we use them to remove gross supragingival calculus deposits as already described.

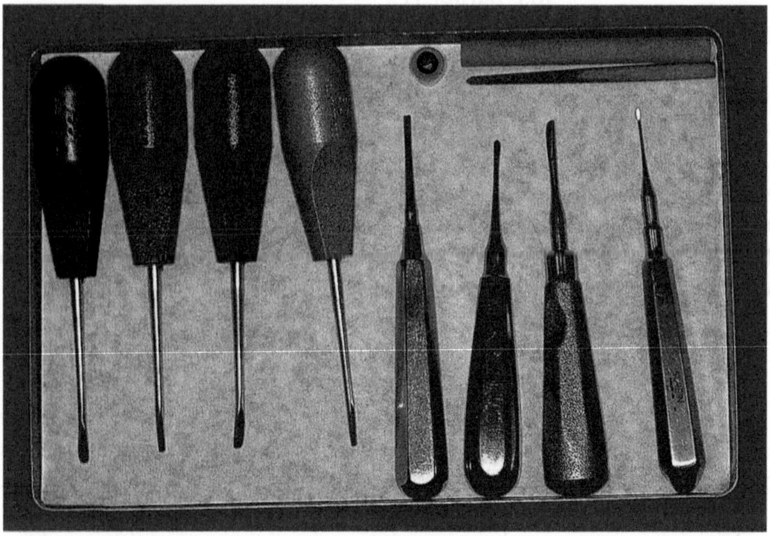

Fig. 2.6 Luxators and elevators. A selection of luxators and elevators are depicted. On the left are four Svensk luxators and on the right four different sizes of Coupland elevators.

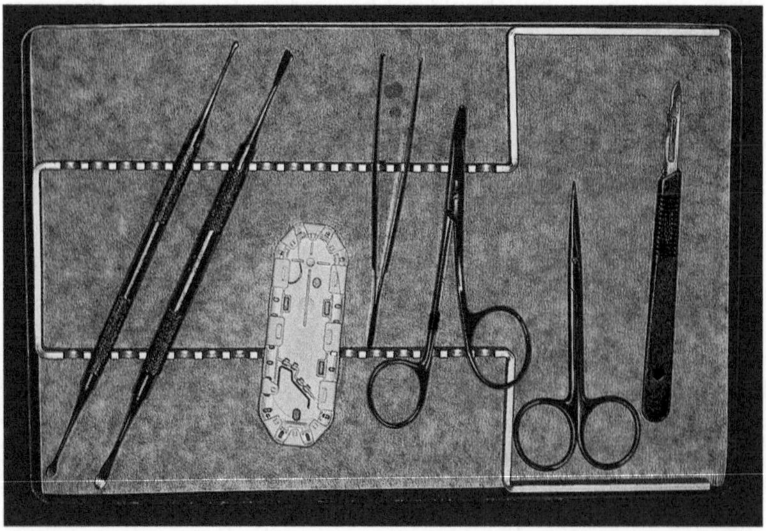

Fig. 2.7 Equipment for tooth extraction. Periosteal elevators and suturing kit (small instruments are required) are depicted. The two periosteal elevators depicted on the left are the Fine P24GSP (for cats) and the Howard P9H (for dogs). Also useful for dogs are the Molt P9 and the Periosteal No. 9.

Scalpel blade

The use of a scalpel blade to free the gingival attachment to the tooth is recommended for both closed and open extraction techniques. A size 15 or 11 blade, used in the handle, is ideal (Fig. 2.7).

Suture kit and suture material

A suture kit with small (ophthalmic) instruments should be available (Fig. 2.7). Always use a monofilament, absorbable suture material in the oral cavity. We currently use Monocryl (poliglecaprone 25, manufactured by Ethicon).

Power equipment

Power equipment is required to perform dentistry and oral surgery. Regular maintenance is essential to avoid problems with equipment failure.

Micromotor unit

A micromotor unit can be used for polishing teeth as well as for sectioning teeth. For sectioning teeth, the micromotor should be set at maximum speed (30 000 rpm). Micromotor units do not generally include water-cooling of the bur and an external source (e.g. assistant applying coolant continuously to the tissues) is required to prevent thermal damage.

Compressed air driven unit

The basic compressed air driven unit consists of a high-speed outlet (which accepts a high-speed handpiece), a slow-speed outlet (which accepts a slow-speed handpiece) and a combination air/water syringe (Fig. 2.9). The high-speed outlet is fitted with water-cooling. The slow-speed outlet may be fitted with water-cooling, but often this feature is absent.

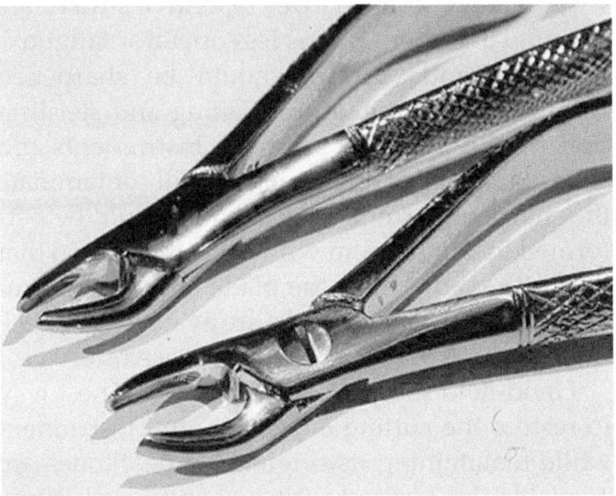

Fig. 2.8 Extraction forceps. Dental forceps are not essential, but if they are to be used then a selection of sizes (to fit the root anatomy of the tooth to be extracted) is required. (Slide courtesy of Big-O, Veterinary Dental Supplies Company.)

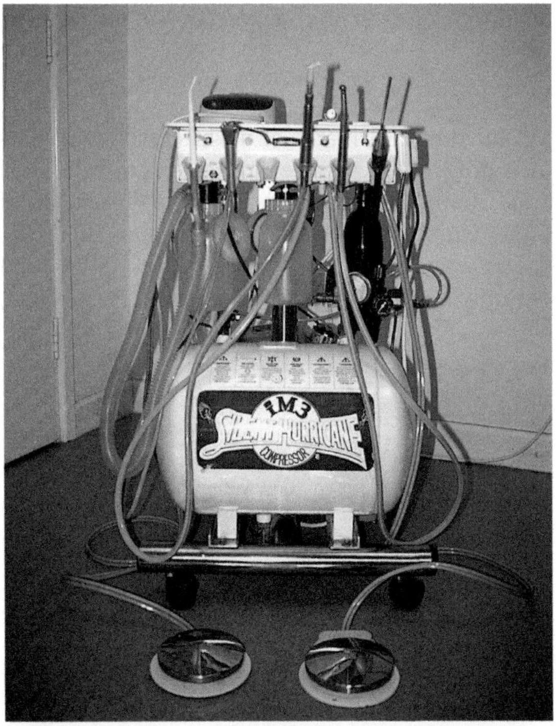

Fig. 2.9 A compressed air driven unit. This compressed air driven unit (iM3), manufactured by Veterinary Instrumentation Ltd, combines a high-speed handpiece (with fibreoptic light), with a slow-speed handpiece and a three-way syringe. It also has the added bonus of suction.

A high-speed handpiece, although not essential for sectioning multirooted teeth prior to extraction, facilitates the process and allows accurate application of coolant water. Investing in a high-speed handpiece with fibreoptic light is strongly recommended.

The slow-speed hand outlet accepts both a contra-angle or straight handpiece. It can be used for sectioning teeth and removing bone (burs) as well as for polishing teeth (prophy cup or brush).

The three-way syringe can deliver either a stream of water or a spray of water and air, or air only. It is used to irrigate/lavage the mouth (water or water/air spray) and to dry the teeth (air only).

Some units come with two high-speed outlets and one of these can be used with a sonic scaler. Suction is also available with some units.

Invest in a compressed air driven unit from the outset. The high-speed handpiece greatly facilitates tooth sectioning and the three-way syringe (for lavage and drying) will aid in the removal of debris and improve visibility. Suction is a real bonus.

Burs

Dental burs are made of a variety of materials including stainless steel, tungsten-carbide steel and 'diamond'. There is a wide selection of burs available to fit both the slow- and the high-speed handpiece (Fig. 2.10). The high-speed handpiece will only accept friction grip burs, while a slow-speed handpiece may accept either friction grip or latch-key burs. A selection of round, pear-shaped, tapered fissure and straight fissure burs will be required for sectioning of teeth and removal of alveolar bone. 'Diamond' burs abrade rather than cut and may be safer for the inexperienced user. Blunted burs should be discarded.

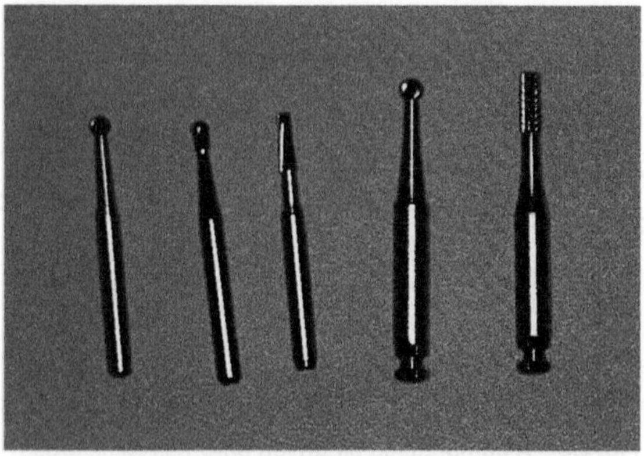

Fig. 2.10 A selection of tungsten carbide burs. From the left are round, pear-shaped and tapered fissure high-speed handpiece burs. Round and cross-cutting straight fissure burs for the slow-speed handpiece are shown on the right.

MISCELLANEOUS

Sharpening

Scalers and curettes, luxators and elevators all require regular sharpening. The basic goals of sharpening are to conserve a sharp cutting edge, and to preserve the original shape of the instrument. Dental instrument sharpening kits (stones and oil), with instructions, are available through veterinary wholesalers. Attending a course to learn how to sharpen instruments is strongly recommended.

Scalers and curettes

Instruments must be sharp if scaling is to be completed efficiently with minimal trauma to the gingival tissues. When the blade of the instrument is maintained properly, greater control of the working end occurs. Fewer repetitive strokes are required and there is thus less operator fatigue.

Scalers and curettes should be sharpened before each use, i.e. after cleaning and sterilisation. Sterilisation will blunt the instruments and sharpening of dirty instruments will contaminate the sharpening stone. Sharpening should be performed in a light room with a bright light, so that the cutting edge(s) of the blade are clearly visualised. Acrylic testing sticks are available to check the adequacy of the sharpening procedure.

Hand-held sharpening stones are the best way to restore the cutting edge on a dull instrument while maintaining its original shape. Stones are available in various grits, shapes and sizes. Coarse stones are used to sharpen very dull instruments, or for reshaping blades. Fine stones will maintain the cutting edge on instruments that are frequently sharpened, without removing an excessive amount of the blade. To prevent 'grooving', the whole surface of the stone should be used during sharpening.

A light mineral oil should be used on the stone. The care of stones involves wiping with a clean cloth to remove metal particles and then scrubbing or ultrasonically cleaning to remove the lubricant. Stones can be autoclaved safely.

There are two basic techniques for instrument sharpening, namely the 'stationary stone, moving instrument' technique or the 'stationary instrument, moving stone' method. The choice of technique depends on operator preference, but the 'stationary instrument, moving stone' method may be easier to learn. Make sure that you are familiar with the component parts of the scaler and curette before attempting sharpening. It may be useful to have a sharp, unused scaler and curette available for comparison during the learning phase. The 'stationary stone, moving instrument' technique for a sickle scaler or universal curette is as follows:

1. Grasp the instrument to be sharpened in your non-dominant hand in a palm grasp and hold the hand against the edge of a counter top.
2. Identify the cutting edge(s) of the instrument.
3. Position the instrument so that the tip or toe of the blade is pointing towards you and the terminal shank is perpendicular to the floor.
4. Spread a thin layer of light mineral oil on the stone; wipe away excess with gauze.
5. Hold the stone in your dominant hand and position the lubricated side against the lateral surface of the blade. Using a clock face as a guide, initially place the stone at a 12 o'clock position.
6. Tilt the top of the stone to slightly less than 1 o'clock (if the stone is held in the left hand, tilt the top of the stone to slightly less than 11 o'clock).
7. Move the stone in a fluid up-and-down motion against the cutting surface, starting at the heel third of the blade and continuing to the tip or toe. You should see a build-up of sludge (oil and metal filings) along the entire facial surface of the blade. Finish your stroke on a downward movement. Remove the sludge and test the sharpness of the cutting edge with an acrylic testing stick.
8. To sharpen the opposite cutting edge, rotate the instrument so that the tip or toe is pointed away from you. Maintain the secure palm grasp and ensure that the terminal shank is perpendicular to the floor. Place the stone at 1 o'clock (11 o'clock if left-handed) and repeat the grinding process. Remove the sludge and test the sharpness of the cutting edge with an acrylic testing stick.
9. To finish a curved sickle scaler or universal curette, place a cylindrical or conical stone on the face of the blade. Lightly rotate the stone along the face from the heel to the tip or toe, applying even pressure.
10. To maintain the rounded shape of the curette toe, rotate the instrument so that the toe is pointed to 3 o'clock. Position the flat stone under the toe and tilt upward toward the 2 o'clock position. Move the stone in a short up-and-down motion, rotating around the toe to maintain the shape.

Each double-ended Gracey curette has an odd and an even number, which identifies the blades. For example, the Gracey 1-2 has the 1 blade on one end and the 2 blade on the opposite end. The procedure for sharpening a Gracey curette using the 'stationary instrument, moving stone' technique is as follows:

1. Hold the instrument in your non-dominant hand with a palm grasp. The odd numbered blade should be at the bottom with the toe facing towards you (point the toe away from you if left-handed). Tilt the terminal shank towards 11 o'clock (1 o'clock if left-handed).
2. Position the lubricated side of the stone against the right lateral surface (left lateral surface if left-handed) and tilt the top of the stone to slightly less than 1 o'clock (11 o'clock if left-handed).
3. Move the stone in a fluid up-and-down motion starting at the heel of the blade and continuing to the toe. Remove the sludge and test the cutting edge with an acrylic testing stick.
4. Now position the instrument so that the even-numbered blade is at the bottom and the toe is pointing away from you (point the toe toward you if left-handed). Repeat the grinding

process keeping the terminal shank at 11 o'clock (1 o'clock if left-handed). Remove the sludge and test the cutting edge with an acrylic testing stick.

Luxators and elevators

Luxators and elevators also need to be sharpened regularly, usually after each use. If the working ends have been damaged, they should be professionally reground.

Luxators and elevators are easily sharpened with a cylindrical Arkansas stone. We prefer to use a 'stationary stone, moving instrument technique' to sharpen these instruments. The technique is as follows:

- Place the cylindrical stone flat on the table
- Spread a thin layer of light mineral oil on the stone; wipe away excess with gauze
- Hold the handle of the luxator or elevator in the palm of the hand, with the index finger extended straight on the shank
- Apply the working end of the luxator or elevator to the stone
- Exert mild pressure and push or pull the luxator and elevator along the stone
- Check sharpness on an acrylic stick
- Repeat as necessary until instrument is sharp

Suction

Suction is invaluable. Excess water and debris can easily be removed, improving visibility for the operator and increasing safety for the patient (reducing the risk of aspiration). In addition, blood loss can be estimated more accurately. Invest in either a compressed air driven unit that incorporates suction (Fig. 2.9) or a separate suction unit.

Care of instruments and equipment

Each patient should receive a clean and sterile set of hand instruments. They are cleaned and sterilised (chemical or heat) in the same fashion as other surgical instruments. Sharpening of scalers, curettes, luxators and elevators can be performed after cleaning, i.e. prior to sterilisation. Heat sterilisation will result in blunting so a clean sharpening stone should be available for sharpening during the procedure. Alternatively, sharpening can be performed after cleaning and sterilisation. The oral cavity is never a sterile site, so while instruments need to be clean, they do not need to be sterile.

Power equipment also requires care and maintenance. The manufacturer and/or supplier of power equipment need to supply you with detailed information about how to care for and maintain the unit that you purchase. An annual service contract should be part of the purchase agreement.

There are similarities and differences in the care and maintenance of different units. The information in the following is a general guide, but you should check with your supplier exactly how your unit should be looked after.

Cleaning and sterilising the ultrasonic scaler

The body of the ultrasonic scaler should not be cleaned in an ultrasonic bath. Instead, it can be cleaned using a cotton swab soaked in alcohol. Following cleaning, the handpiece should be sterilised (autoclaving at 134°C at 2 bar (200 kPa) for 20 minutes). The procedure is as follows:

- Separate the handpiece from the cord and remove the scaler tip
- Put the handpiece in the sterilisable cloth or bag if required
- Take the handpiece out of the autoclave as soon as the sterilisation is complete
- Carefully dry the electrical contacts of the handpiece and the cord connector before use

Cleaning and sterilising handpieces

Handpieces (contra-angle and high-speed) should be cleaned, sterilised and lubricated after each operation. Each patient should receive clean and sterile instruments and this includes handpieces.

Handpieces need to be lubricated after cleaning, i.e. prior to sterilisation. They then need to be lubricated again after sterilisation, i.e. prior to use. Handpieces need to be lubricated before and after sterilisation or the bearings will fail. They should be sterilised by autoclaving. Dry heat sterilisation should not be used.

Important points relating to the high-speed handpiece are:

- Ensure that the water switch is in the 'On' position
- Do not operate if there is insufficient water in the bottle
- It should never be operated without a bur inserted

After removing the bur, a brush is used to remove foreign particles from the handpiece. It is then wiped clean with a moist cloth. For the high-speed handpiece, a fine wire is provided for cleaning the water spray hole. Instructions should come with each unit as to how to dismantle handpieces. Read these instructions carefully.

Lubricate the handpiece. This can be achieved by inserting two to three drops of oil lubricant via a lubricant nozzle into the air supply tube. If a spray lubricant is used, it should be activated for 3 seconds. Operate handpiece with bur installed for 15–20 seconds. Remove bur from the handpiece and disconnect the handpiece from the unit. The handpiece is now ready for autoclaving. Follow the manufacturer's directions. After autoclaving is complete, make sure the handpiece returns to room temperature and lubricate it again prior to use. Lack of lubrication will cause malfunction.

Cautions

- Never autoclave handpiece with bur in place
- Never operate handpiece without bur inserted
- Do not forget 'before and after sterilisation' lubrication procedures
- Dry heat sterilisation is not allowed under any circumstances

General maintenance

Table 2.1 indicates general maintenance required for power equipment.

Important: The high-speed handpiece requires clean air, and water that accumulates in the compressor must be removed daily. Refer to the handbook for details of how to empty the compressor.

Table 2.1 General maintenance requirements

Operation	Daily	Weekly	Annually
Drain air receiver	★		
Drain filter/regulator	★		
Check oil level		★	
Change oil			★
Change air intake filter			★
Change line filter			★
Check electrical connections and all pipe fittings			★

Summary

- Dental procedures require a designated room or area designed to facilitate safe and effective clinical working practices
- Face masks and eye protection for operator and assistant are important
- Clean, preferably sterile instruments should be available for each patient
- Have ready-made 'kits' available for different procedures, e.g. periodontal therapy, extraction etc
- Sharpen instruments (e.g. scalers, curettes, luxators, elevators, etc.) before each use, i.e. after cleaning and sterilisation
- Regular maintenance of power equipment is essential
- Lubricate all handpieces on the dental unit prior to use. They should also be oiled prior to sterilisation
- When autoclaving the handpieces, always remove the bur
- Never operate handpiece without bur inserted

FURTHER READING

Gorrel, C. & Penman, S. (1995) Dental equipment. In: Crossley, D. & Penman, S. (eds) *Manual of Small Animal Dentistry*. Cheltenham: BSAVA, Ch. 2, pp. 12–26.

Smarten up, Sharpen Up. A Practical Workbook on Sharpening Dental Curets and Scalers. Chicago: Hu-Friedy Inc., 1982.

Verstraete, F.J.M. (ed) (1999) *Self-assessment Colour Review of Veterinary Dentistry*. London: Manson.

Wiggs, R.B. & Lobprise, H.B. (1997) Dental equipment. In Wiggs, R.B. & Lobprise, H.B. (eds) *Veterinary Dentistry: Principles and Practice*. Philadelphia: Lippincott-Raven, Ch. 1, pp. 1–28.

3

Anaesthetic monitoring and immediate postoperative care

A full clinical examination of the oral cavity and all oral procedures require general anaesthesia. Anaesthesia is an unnatural state, and the induction of anaesthesia always carries a risk. While the anaesthetic mortality rate in fit and healthy cats and dogs is 1 in 679 (0.15%), it increases to around 1 in 31 (3.2%) in animals that have disease (Clarke & Hall, 1990). In a more recent study (Dyson et al, 1998) investigating the morbidity and mortality associated with anaesthesia (8087 dogs and 8702 cats), the incidences of complications were 2.1% in dogs and 0.13% in cats and the mortality rate was 0.11% in dogs and 0.1% in cats. Among other factors, continuous monitoring of anaesthesia was associated with reduced mortality.

This chapter will cover anaesthetic monitoring and postoperative care for the patient undergoing dental treatment and/or oral surgery. The legal status of the veterinary nurse and technician varies from country to country. In the UK, veterinary nurses may do the things specified in paragraphs 6 (applies to listed veterinary nurses) and 7 (applies to student veterinary nurses) of Schedule 3 to the Veterinary Surgeons Act 1966, as amended by the Veterinary Surgeons Act 1966 (Schedule 3 Amendment) Order 2002, SI 2002/1479, with effect from 10 June 2002. See Appendix 1 for full text.

GENERAL PRINCIPLES OF ANAESTHESIA FOR THE DENTAL PATIENT

Airway security

During dental surgery, the airway must be secured by endotracheal intubation to prevent aspiration pneumonia, which may occur if debris (irrigation fluid, blood) from the oral cavity enters unprotected airways. This condition may be fatal and is easier to prevent than to cure.

Endotracheal tubes

Endotracheal tubes must be checked for defective cuffs and obstructed lumens before use. Any defective tubes should be discarded. Lightweight circuits are recommended.

To reduce apparatus dead space and the risk of endobronchial intubation, the tubing should be cut to fit the patient from midneck to the level of the incisor teeth. Excessively long tubes that protrude from the oral cavity are prone to kinking, which may lead to pulmonary oedema as the patient inspires against an obstructed airway. The use of guarded endotracheal tubes should be considered for patients at high risk of tube kinking. Moreover, excessively long tubes are difficult to secure to the jaw with gauze bandage, which increases the risk of accidental extubation. Knots should be tied around the adapter and not around the endotracheal tube itself. The cuff should be carefully inflated to a point where there is no air leaking around it. Be careful not to inflate the cuff excessively as this can cause tracheal injury. The status of the endotracheal tube and integrity of the cuff should be monitored continuously. The operator will usually change the animal's position during surgery or while taking radiographs and this may cause tube displacement and/or kinking. If the surgical site is draped, the drapes need to be lifted at regular intervals to assess endotracheal tube status.

Pharyngeal packing

Pharyngeal packing should be used for greater airway security. Commonly used pharyngeal packs include surgical swabs, sponges and gauze bandage. A simple way to pack the pharynx is to insert a length of damp gauze bandage around the endotracheal tube with the free end left visible for easy removal. It is important not to pack too tightly as this impedes venous return and results in swelling of the tongue. Packs will become saturated with liquid during procedures. They will then no longer offer adequate protection and should be replaced as required. It is imperative to remove any packing prior to extubation.

Eye protection

The eyes should be protected from desiccation by applying a lubricant eye ointment as required during the procedure.

Mouth gags

Mouth gags should be used with caution. Keeping the jaws wide open for prolonged periods may result in neuropraxia and inability to close the jaws. The condition is self-limiting but may take several weeks to resolve. Mouth gags should be released and the jaws closed every 10–15 minutes. Keeping a record of how long the mouth gag has been in place ensures that the jaws are not inadvertently kept wide open for more than 15 minutes.

Suction

It is recommended to use suction to protect the airways from saliva, irrigation fluids and other debris. In addition, blood loss can also be estimated by measuring the volume of blood in the suction jar.

Long anaesthetic periods

Dental procedures are often lengthy and close attention to life support is needed:

- Oxygen should be delivered at an inspired concentration of at least 33% to compensate for the deterioration in pulmonary function that accompanies anaesthesia even in healthy young patients
- Reduced cardiac output and arterial blood pressure produced by anaesthesia should be offset by intravenous fluid therapy
- Hypothermia is a complication of lengthy anaesthesia and the use of cool irrigation fluids. Hypothermia results in anticholinergic resistant bradycardia, reduced cardiac output and haemoconcentration. Cardiac fibrillation can occur at a body temperature of around 28°C. Moreover, requirements for anaesthetic agents are reduced during hypothermia and care should be taken to prevent relative overdose. Body temperature should be monitored regularly, e.g. every 20–30 minutes, and the development of hypothermia should be prevented by supplying external heat by blankets and warmed intravenous and irrigation fluids. Patients should be insulated with towels or bubble pack to prevent thermal injuries due to 'hot spots' that may occur with electrical heating mats. Circulating warm water mats may be safer
- Hyperthermia can occasionally occur in large heavy-coated dogs connected to rebreathing circuits for long periods. By monitoring body temperature every 20–30 minutes, the development of hyperthermia can be identified and active cooling (fans, cooling pads, etc.) can be initiated before damage occurs to vital organs

Haemorrhage

Periodontal and other dental treatments rarely result in extensive haemorrhage unless the patient has an underlying disorder, i.e. coagulopathy, septicaemia.

A full haematological examination and clotting profile should be performed prior to any potentially haemorrhagic procedure, e.g. major oral surgery such as a maxillectomy. The patient should also be cross-matched with a healthy donor prior to any such procedure. An alternative to cross-matching is autologous transfusion where one week before surgery 10% of the patient's blood volume is removed and replaced with intravenous fluids. The blood is stored at 4°C in acid-citrate-dextrose or citrate-phosphate-dextrose transfusion packs until required.

During the procedure, blood loss should be estimated either by weighing blood-soaked swabs or by measuring the amount of blood collected in a suction jar. As a rough guide a saturated 3 × 3 inch swab contains 7 ml of blood and a saturated 4 × 4 inch swab contains 10 ml of blood.

PATIENT MONITORING

All patients should be monitored continuously. Careful monitoring should enable the detection of problems before they become severe, so that they can be treated appropriately and crises can be avoided. As already mentioned, continuous anaesthetic monitoring is associated with reduced mortality (Dyson et al, 1998). It is impossible to both monitor anaesthesia and perform the procedure. Moreover, with some procedures a surgical assistant is required. The surgical assistant needs to be a different person from the one monitoring the anaesthesia.

Prior to the induction of anaesthesia, the anaesthetic machine must be checked to ensure that it is functioning properly and that oxygen, nitrous oxide (if used) and volatile agents (isoflurane or halothane) levels are adequate. Routine anaesthetic monitoring includes:

- Inspecting respiratory function
- Assessing the colour of the mucous membranes
- Checking capillary refill time
- Listening to the sound of breathing
- Palpating the peripheral pulse

All findings should be recorded on an anaesthetic chart at regular intervals, e.g. every 5 or 10 minutes, during the duration of anaesthesia (Fig. 3.1). Also record current oxygen, nitrous oxide (if used) and volatile agent level at each check. Any changes in the anaesthetic regimen, e.g. altering flow rate or concentration of volatile agent, should be recorded on the chart. Remember to check the levels of the cylinders and vaporisers at regular intervals.

This basic monitoring can be augmented with mechanical aids, which give additional information and allow a more precise picture of the patient's status. This allows closer control over the course of the anaesthetic. The disadvantage of mechanical monitoring devices is that they in turn must be monitored to ensure that the information they are giving is accurate. Unexpected readings should be verified by examination of the patient before they are acted on, i.e. monitor the patient, not the equipment.

Monitoring checklist

- Endotracheal tube is correctly positioned and the cuff is not overinflated
- Endotracheal tube is securely fastened and not kinked
- Accidental extubation or circuit disconnection has not occurred (apnoea alarms and capnograms are useful for detecting accidental disconnection)
- Monitor the central nervous system (ocular signs and muscle tone will indicate the depth of anaesthesia)
- Monitor the cardiovascular system (pulse quality, auscultation of heart sounds, mucous membrane colour and capillary refill). Monitoring devices that aid clinical assessment of cardiovascular function include oesophageal stethoscopes, blood pressure monitors and electrocardiogram (ECG)
- Monitor the respiratory system (tidal volume assessment by observing the rebreathing bag and chest wall excursions, respiratory rate, and mucous membrane colour). Monitoring devices include apnoea alarms and pulse oximeters
- Monitor and record body temperature (rectal or oesophageal)
- Monitor renal function (a urinary catheter connected to an empty intravenous fluid bag via an administration set can measure urine output and thus give an indication of organ perfusion)
- Estimate blood loss
- Replace saturated pharyngeal packs
- Release mouth gags at regular intervals
- Reapply eye ointment as required

WEIGHT	kg		
PREMED	Acp	Atropine	Vetergesic
INDUCTION	Rapinovet		
OTHER			

DATE:------------------------- PATIENT NAME:----------------------------------

OWNER NAME:----------------------------------

START TIME:------------------ FINISH TIME:-------------------------------------

Time									
Resp									
Pulse									
CRT									
O_2									
Iso									
Temp									

Fig. 3.1 An example of a basic anaesthetic chart. Acp = acepromazine; CRT = capillary refill time; Iso = isoflurane.

Many of the patients that require dental procedures are geriatric. It must be remembered that even clinically healthy geriatric patients have physiological changes in the cardiopulmonary system that can influence the course of anaesthesia. Important age-related changes include:

- Decreased cardiac output
- Reduced ability to compensate for blood pressure and circulating volume changes
- Decreased lung compliance
- High small airway closing volume
- Decreased partial pressure of oxygen in arterial blood (PaO_2)

A noticeable decrease in circulation time is seen during induction, and further increments of injectable anaesthetic agents should not be given too soon.

In addition to the age-related physiological changes, elderly patients also have psychological requirements in that they are easily distressed and confused by changes in routine and require gentle handling and constant reassurance.

ANAESTHETIC RECOVERY

Anaesthesia should be lightened towards the end of the procedure. The oral cavity must be cleaned, the pharyngeal pack removed and the cuff of the endotracheal tube deflated before recovery is allowed to proceed. Use of the three-way syringe (air–water spray) on the dental unit is recommended for removing debris from the tongue and gums. A dry swab can be used to remove any large blood clots. Ensure that there is no debris in the oropharynx before removing the pharyngeal pack and deflating the cuff of the endotracheal tube. The coat around the mouth and head should be cleaned and dried (towel and hairdryer). Recovery should always occur in a warm environment.

The endotracheal tube is usually not removed until the animal has a swallowing reflex.

Anaesthetic recovery should be monitored closely and recorded. Animals that have had surgical procedures using flap techniques and suturing, e.g. open (surgical) extractions or oronasal fistula repair, need to be prevented from pawing at their mouth or rubbing their faces. In some animals, an Elizabethan collar may need to be fitted. If the surgical procedure has resulted in blood in the nasal cavity, e.g. oronasal fistula repair, it is wise to recover these patients in sternal recumbency with the head placed lower than the rest of the body to encourage drainage. Sneezing fits commonly occur on recovery with these patients.

IMMEDIATE POSTOPERATIVE CARE

Optimal immediate postoperative management involves appropriate analgesia and nursing. Long-term postoperative care for the dental patient is usually a combination of professional intervention and home care (measures taken by the owner to remove or reduce plaque accumulation on a daily basis). Home care is essential. It is covered in Chapter 10.

ANALGESIA

Humans can express and describe the sensations of discomfort and/or pain that they experience, and these descriptions are well accepted. Assessment of pain in animals is much more difficult. One must rely on overt signs and the correct interpretation of these signs. Animals probably have no psychological expectation of pain, so the confounding influence of anticipation is removed. Changed responsiveness to human contact is often a first indicator that the animal is in discomfort. Aggression or avoidance of human contact may occur, but some animals seek excessive human reassurance. Disturbance in the sleep pattern, with an animal sleeping less, is also an indicator of discomfort. Reduced grooming and changes in eating behaviour are often manifestations of chronic pain. In the presence of oral/dental disease it is rare for the animal to stop eating, instead they change their food preferences (e.g. an animal will selectively only eat soft food) or change the way they chew (e.g. chew selectively on one side). A common feedback from clients after their pet has undergone a remedial dental procedure is that the animal is brighter in general, often showing more interest in exercise and games than prior to treatment. One can speculate that this commonly reported change in general behaviour is attributable to the removal of chronic discomfort and pain.

In human dentistry, there is a good understanding of which disease processes cause discomfort and pain. We also know which procedures are associated with postoperative pain. It seems reasonable to assume that dogs and cats experience discomfort and pain when afflicted by the same diseases and after receiving similar treatment. In following this line of reasoning, overtreatment with analgesics may occur, but the adverse consequences of this are minimal compared with the distress of withholding pain relief.

Common conditions that we know are likely to cause discomfort and/or pain in people and are thus likely to cause similar sensations to an affected animal include:

1. Complications to periodontitis, e.g. lateral periodontal abscess, toxic mucous membrane ulcers, gingivostomatitis
2. Pulp and periapical disease, e.g. acute pulpitis, periapical abscess, osteomyelitis
3. Traumatic injuries, including soft tissue lacerations and jaw fracture.

Dental procedures that are associated with postoperative pain in humans, and are therefore likely to do the same in animals, include:

1. Periodontal therapy, e.g. deep subgingival curettage
2. Extraction, especially when extraction sockets are left to heal by granulation

Pain should be prevented rather than simply treated. The concept of pre-emptive analgesia is the administration of analgesics preoperatively to reduce the severity of postoperative pain. However, pre-emptive analgesia does not eliminate postoperative pain, so additional measures are still required to ensure a comfortable recovery.

A basic analgesic routine, which can be modified as required, is shown in the box.

Basic dental analgesic plan

- An opioid is included in the premedication
- Additional opioid is given intraoperatively or local anaesthetics are administered prior to starting the surgical procedure
- Opioids and/or non-steroidal anti-inflammatory drugs (NSAIDs) are administered postoperatively. Local anaesthesia (administered at the end of a procedure) will also provide postoperative analgesia
- NSAIDs are used during recovery

NURSING

Sound nursing measures also have a profound impact on reducing the level of postoperative discomfort and pain.

A quiet environment allowing the animal to sleep is most important. The intensity of acute postoperative pain generally diminishes quickly. Sleeping it off is beneficial! Cats, in particular, appreciate a quiet environment postoperatively; a barking dog in the same room is not conducive to a stress-free recovery.

Giving the animal attention at regular intervals helps reduce the distress associated with pain and the unfamiliar environment; otherwise a cycle of pain/distress/sleeplessness can develop.

The provision of a comfortable bed in a warm, but not too hot, environment is beneficial. Food and water should be offered as early as possible in the postoperative period. Pain and inflammation increase the basic metabolic rate and a high level of nutrition is required to promote healing. Offering food as early as possible not only speeds recovery, but can also have a soothing effect.

Summary

- Most dental treatment requires general anaesthesia, and standard good clinical practice should be followed
- During dental surgery the airway must be secured by endotracheal intubation
- Pharyngeal packing must be available for each patient. It is imperative that it is removed prior to extubation
- Mouth gags should be used with caution
- Attention should be given to maintaining body temperature and fluid balance
- All patients should be monitored continuously, and findings recorded on a chart
- Monitor recovery closely
- Good nursing promotes good recovery

REFERENCES

Clark, K.W. & Hall, L.W. (1990) A survey of anaesthesia in small animal practice: AVA/BSAVA report. *Journal of the Association of Veterinary Anaesthesia* **17**: 4–10.

Dyson, D.H., Maxie, M.G. & Schnurr, D. (1998) Morbidity and mortality associated with anesthetic management in small animal veterinary practice in Ontario. *Journal of the American Animal Hospital Association* **34**(4): 325–335.

4

Anatomy of the teeth and periodontium

The dentition of dogs and cats resembles that of humans. There are differences in tooth number and shape, but the basic anatomy is similar. The dentition of rodents and lagomorphs is covered in Chapter 12.

Each tooth has a crown (above the gum) and one or more roots (below the gum). The bulk of the mature tooth is composed of dentine, which is covered by enamel on the crown and by cementum on the roots. The centre of the tooth contains the pulp or endodontic system. Figure 4.1 depicts the basic structure of a tooth.

The crowns of dog and cat teeth have a more tapered shape with sharp cutting edges and fewer chewing surfaces as compared to human teeth. Also the teeth are spaced further apart and where there is contact between teeth, the contact area is smaller and not as tight as in humans.

Humans, dogs and cats are diphyodont, i.e. primary (deciduous) teeth are followed by a permanent dentition. Dental formulae describe the type and number of teeth in each quadrant. 'I' represents incisor teeth, 'C' represents canine teeth, 'P' represents premolars and 'M' represents molars. The respective dental formulae of the primary and permanent dentitions of dog and cat are shown in the box.

The formation of the crown of both primary and permanent teeth occurs while a tooth is developing within the alveolar bone. Enamel formation is completed before the tooth erupts into the oral cavity. Once the enamel has formed, the

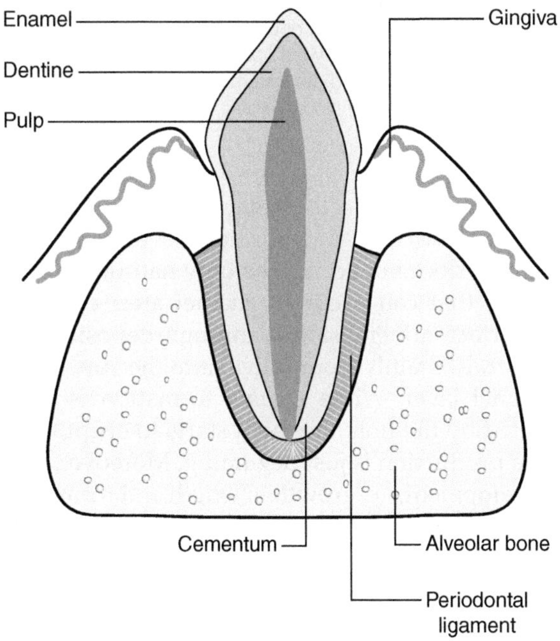

Fig. 4.1 Basic anatomy of the tooth and the periodontium.

Dental formulae for cats and dogs

Dog:
Primary teeth: 2 × {I 3/3 : C 1/1 : P 3/3} = 28
Permanent teeth: 2 × {I 3/3 : C 1/1 : P 4/4 : M 2/3} = 42

Cat:
Primary teeth: 2 × {I 3/3 : C 1/1 : P 3/2} = 26
Permanent teeth: 2 × {I 3/3 : C 1/1 : P 3/2 : M 1/1} = 30

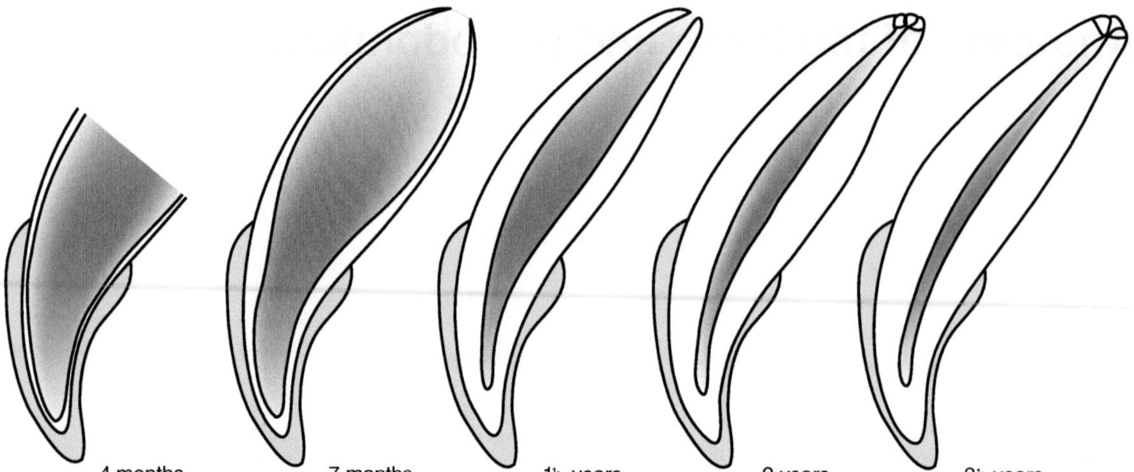

Fig. 4.2 Maturation of a permanent canine tooth after eruption. Enamel formation is complete at the time of eruption, while dentine production and root development (root elongation and formation of an apex) are just beginning. The apical foramen of an immature tooth is a single wide opening. As the individual ages, closure of the apex (apexogenesis) occurs by continuous deposition of dentine and cementum until, in mature teeth, the root apex consists of numerous small openings or foramina allowing the passage of blood vessels, lymphatics and nerves.

ameloblasts (the cells that produce the enamel matrix) are lost and further development of enamel does not occur. The only natural form of repair that can occur to enamel after eruption is surface mineralisation, through deposition of minerals, mainly from saliva, into the superficial enamel layer. While enamel formation is completed by the time the tooth starts to erupt, dentine production is just beginning. Moreover, root development, i.e. growth in length and formation of a root apex, is by no means complete at the time of eruption. Figure 4.2 depicts maturation of a permanent tooth following eruption.

The primary teeth start forming in utero and erupt between 3 and 12 weeks of age. The permanent crowns start forming at, or shortly after, birth and mineralisation of the crowns is complete by around 11 weeks of age. Resorption and exfoliation of the primary teeth and replacement by the permanent dentition occurs between 3 and 7 months of age in the dog and between 3 and 5 months of age in the cat. Once the crowns of the permanent teeth have erupted, root development continues for several months. The approximate ages when teeth erupt in dogs and cats are shown in Table. 4.1.

Table 4.1 Approximate ages (in weeks) when teeth erupt in dogs and cats

	Primary teeth		Permanent teeth	
	Puppy	Kitten	Dog	Cat
Incisors	4–6	3–4	12–16	11–16
Canines	3–5	3–4	12–16	12–20
Premolars	5–6	5–6	16–20	16–20
Molars	–	–	16–24	20–24

ANATOMY OF THE TOOTH

As already mentioned, the tooth consists of enamel, dentine, cementum and pulp. The detailed structure of these tissues will be discussed below.

Enamel

Enamel is the hardest and most mineralised tissue in the body. It does not have a nerve or a blood supply. The inorganic content of mature enamel amounts to 96–97% of the weight, the remainder being organic material and water (Fejerskov & Thylstrup, 1979). The inorganic material consists of calcium hydroxyapatite crystals arranged in an orderly fashion at right angles to the tooth surface. The organic content is made up of soluble and insoluble proteins and peptides.

The enamel of dog and cat teeth is thinner than that of human teeth, generally being 0.2 mm in the cat and 0.5 mm in dogs, and rarely exceeding 1 mm even at the tips of the teeth (Crossley, 1995). This compares with a thickness of up to 2.5 mm in humans (Schroeder, 1991).

Dentine

The bulk of the mature tooth is made up of dentine, which is continuously deposited throughout life by odontoblasts lining the pulp system. The primary dentine is the first layer that forms. It is the dentine that is present at the time of tooth eruption. Throughout life there is a slow continuous physiological deposition of dentine, which is called secondary dentine. In response to trauma, dentine is laid down rapidly and in a less organised fashion. This type of dentine is called reparative or tertiary dentine.

The composition of dentine on a wet weight basis is 70% inorganic material, 18% organic material and 12% water (Mjör, 1979). The inorganic portion of dentine consists mainly of calcium hydroxyapatite crystals similar to those seen in cementum and bone, but smaller than the hydroxyapatite crystals seen in enamel. The organic portion consists mainly of collagen.

Dentine has a tubular structure. Dentinal tubules make up 20 to 30% of the volume of dentine. The tubules traverse the entire width of the dentine, from the pulpal tissue to the dentino-enamel junction (DEJ) in the crown or the dentino-cementum junction (DCJ) in the root. They contain the cytoplasmic processes of the odontoblasts and dentinal fluid. The dentine tubules are more numerous and have a wider diameter closer to the pulp than towards the enamel or cementum surface. The number of dentine tubules (20 000–40 000/mm^2) and diameter (tapering from 3–4 μm near the pulp to under 1 μm in the outer layer of dentine) is similar in cats, dogs, monkeys and humans (Forssell-Ahlberg et al, 1975).

Cementum

Cementum, although part of the tooth, is classified as part of the periodontium and is discussed later in this chapter.

Pulp

The pulp is composed of connective tissue liberally interspersed with tiny blood vessels, lymphatics, myelinated and unmyelinated nerves and undifferentiated mesenchymal cells. As already mentioned, the pulp system is lined by odontoblasts, which produce dentine.

In the crown, the section containing the pulp is called the pulp chamber and in the root(s), it is called the root canal(s). The root canal opens into the periapical tissues at the root apex. The apical foramen of immature teeth is a single wide opening. As the individual ages, closure of the apex (apexogenesis) occurs by continuous deposition of dentine and cementum (Fig. 4.2) until, in mature teeth, the root apex consists of numerous small openings or foramina allowing the passage of blood vessels, lymphatics and nerves.

ANATOMY OF THE PERIODONTIUM

The periodontium is an anatomical unit which functions to attach the tooth to the jaw and provide a suspensory apparatus resilient to normal functional forces. It is made up of gingiva, periodontal ligament, cementum and alveolar bone (Fig. 4.1).

The gingiva

The gingiva surrounds the teeth and the marginal parts of the alveolar bone, forming a cuff around each tooth.

The gingiva (Figs 4.3 and 4.4) can be divided into the free gingiva, which is closely adapted to the tooth surface, and the attached gingiva, which is firmly attached to the underlying periosteum of the alveolar bone. The attached gingiva is delineated from the oral mucosa by the mucogingival line, except in the palate where no such delineation exists. An interdental papilla is

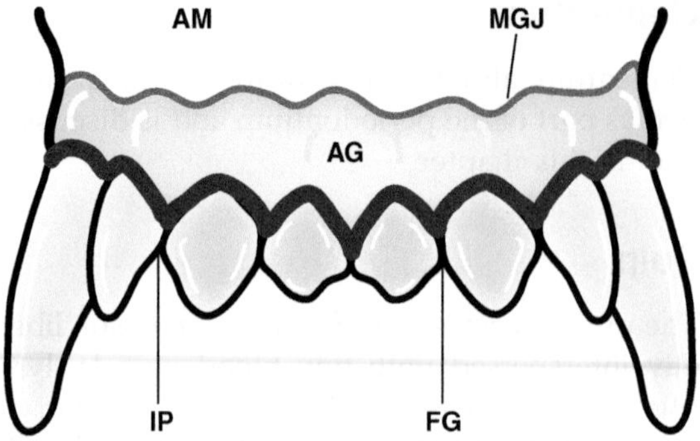

Fig. 4.3 The visible landmarks of clinically normal gingiva. MGJ = mucogingival junction or line; AM = alveolar mucosa; AG = attached gingiva; FG = free gingiva; IP = interdental papilla.

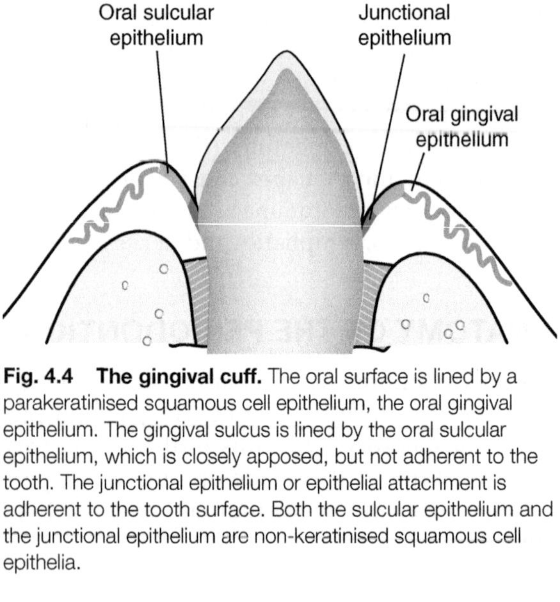

Fig. 4.4 The gingival cuff. The oral surface is lined by a parakeratinised squamous cell epithelium, the oral gingival epithelium. The gingival sulcus is lined by the oral sulcular epithelium, which is closely apposed, but not adherent to the tooth. The junctional epithelium or epithelial attachment is adherent to the tooth surface. Both the sulcular epithelium and the junctional epithelium are non-keratinised squamous cell epithelia.

formed by the gingival tissues in the spaces between the teeth (the interproximal spaces).

The margin of the free gingiva is rounded in such a way that a small invagination or sulcus is formed between the tooth and the gingiva. Therefore, the gingival sulcus is a shallow groove surrounding each tooth. The depth of the sulcus can be assessed by gently inserting a graduated periodontal probe until resistance is encountered. This resistance is taken to be the base of the sulcus. The depth from the free gingival margin to the base of the sulcus can thus be measured

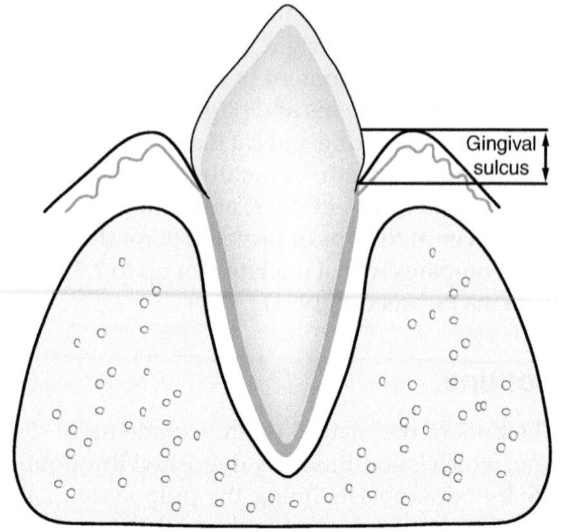

Fig. 4.5 The gingival sulcus. The gingival sulcus is measured from the free gingival margin to the base of the sulcus.

(Fig. 4.5). In the periodontally healthy individual, the sulcus is 1–3 mm deep in humans and dogs and 0.5–1 mm in cats.

The oral surface of the gingiva is lined by a parakeratinised squamous cell epithelium, the oral gingival epithelium. The gingival sulcus is lined by the oral sulcular epithelium. In addition to the sulcular epithelium, which is closely apposed to the tooth surface but not attached, there is a thin layer of highly permeable epithelium which is adherent to the tooth surface called the epithelial attachment or junctional epithelium. Both the oral sulcular epithelium and the junctional epithelium are non-keratinised squamous cell epithelia and have a very rapid cell turnover (5–8 days).

The gingival connective tissue is densely fibrous and firmly attached to the periosteum of the alveolar bone.

Periodontal ligament

The periodontal ligament is the connective tissue that attaches the root cementum to the alveolar bone. It acts as a suspensory ligament for the tooth, and is in a continual state of physiological activity.

The collagen fibres within the ligament are arranged in functional groups. Individual fibres do not span the entire distance between bone and cementum; they branch and reunite in an interwoven pattern. All fibres follow a wavy course that allows for slight movement of the tooth and will absorb mild impact to the tooth.

Cementum

The cementum is an avascular bone-like tissue that covers the root surface. It does not contain Haversian canals and is therefore denser than bone. It is less calcified than enamel or dentine; but like dentine, cementum deposition is continuous throughout life. Cementum is a very important component involved in tooth support, as it is capable of both resorptive and reparative processes. Resorption and apposition are, however, slower than in bone.

Alveolar bone

The alveolar bone is composed of the ridges of the jaw that support the teeth. The roots of the teeth are contained in deep depressions, the alveolar sockets in the bone. The alveolar bone develops during tooth eruption and undergoes atrophy with tooth loss. It responds readily to external and systemic influences. The usual response to stimuli results in resorption, but this may be accompanied by apposition in some situations.

Alveolar bone consists of four layers. In addition to the three layers found in all bones, namely periosteum, dense compact bone and cancellous bone, there is a fourth layer called the cribriform plate, which lines the alveolar sockets. Radiographically, this appears as a fine radiodense line called the lamina dura. The margin of the crest of alveolar bone is normally located around 1 mm below the cemento-enamel junction. Vessels and nerves run through the alveolar bone and perforate the cribriform plate. The majority of these blood and nerve vessels supply the periodontal ligament.

Summary

- Cats and dogs (like humans) are diphyodont, i.e. primary (deciduous) teeth are shed to make way for the permanent dentition
- The bulk of the mature tooth is composed of dentine, covered by enamel on the crown and cementum on the roots
- Enamel is the hardest tissue in the body, consisting mainly of calcium hydroxyapatite. Its formation is complete by the time of tooth eruption. Regeneration is not possible, only repair by surface mineralisation
- The endodontic system (pulp) makes up the centre of the tooth and contains odontoblasts, which produce dentine throughout the life of the animal
- The periodontium serves to support the tooth and absorb functional forces. It consists of the gingiva, periodontal ligament, cementum and alveolar bone

REFERENCES

Crossley, D.A. (1995) Results of a preliminary study of enamel thickness in the mature dentition of domestic dogs and cats. *Journal of Veterinary Dentistry* **12**(3): 111–113.

Fejerskov, O. & Thylstrup, A. (1979) Dental enamel. In: Mjör, I.A. & Fejerskov, O. (eds) *Histology of the Human Tooth*, 2nd edn. Copenhagen: Munksgaard, pp. 75–103.

Forssell-Ahlberg, K., Brännström, M. & Edwall, L. (1975) The diameter and number of dentinal tubules in rat, cat, dog and monkey. A comparative scanning electron microscope study. *Acta Odontologica Scandinavica* **33**: 234–250.

Mjör, I.A. (1979) Dentin and pulp. In: Mjör, I.A. & Fejerskov, O. (eds) *Histology of the Human Tooth*, 2nd edn. Copenhagen: Munksgaard, pp. 43–74.

Schroeder, H.E. (1991) *Oral Structural Biology*. New York: Thieme.

5

Occlusion and malocclusion

Occlusion is defined as the normal position of the teeth when the jaws are closed.

In normal occlusion the length and width of the jaws and the position of the teeth in the respective jaws are in harmony.

The development of the occlusion is determined primarily by genetic factors. It is known that jaw length, tooth bud position and tooth size are inherited (Stockard, 1941). It is also known that the development of the upper jaw, mandible and teeth are independently regulated genetically (Stockard, 1941).

Malocclusion is an abnormality in the position of the teeth. It is common in dogs, but also occurs in cats. The development of malocclusion is determined by both genetic and environmental factors. Malocclusion can result from jaw length and/or width discrepancy (skeletal malocclusion), from tooth malpositioning (dental malocclusion) or a combination of both. Specific genetic mechanisms regulating malocclusion are unknown. A polygenic mechanism, however, is likely and explains why not all siblings in successive generations are affected by malocclusion to the same degree, if affected at all. With a polygenic mechanism, the severity of clinical signs is linked to the number of defective genes.

The most reasonable approach suggested (Hennet & Harvey, 1992; Hennet, 1995) to evaluate whether malocclusion is hereditary or acquired is as follows:

- Skeletal malocclusion is considered inherited unless a developmental cause can be reliably identified
- Pure dental malocclusion, unless known to have breed or family predisposition, should be given the benefit of doubt and not be considered inherited

NORMAL OCCLUSION

When evaluating occlusion it is important to look at all parameters and not to base judgement solely on the positioning of the incisor teeth. In fact, the canine and premolar relationships often give a better guide to the occlusion.

The shape of the head affects the positioning of the teeth. Malocclusion occurs in any of the three head shapes (dolicocephalic, mesocephalic and brachycephalic), but is more common in brachycephalic breeds.

Dog

In the mesocephalic dog, the mandible is shorter and less wide than the upper jaw. The normal bite of the adult mesocephalic dog is characterised by the following features.

Scissor bite of the incisor teeth (Fig. 5.1)

- The upper incisors are rostral to the lower incisors

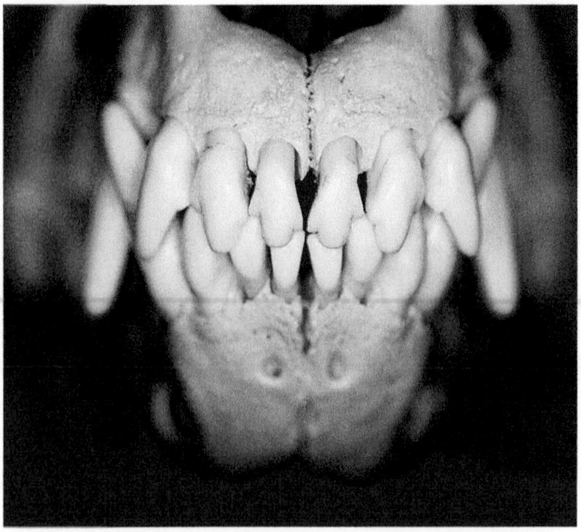

Fig. 5.1 Scissor bite of the incisor teeth. The upper incisors are rostral to the lower, with the incisal tips of the mandibular incisors contacting the cingulae of the upper incisors.

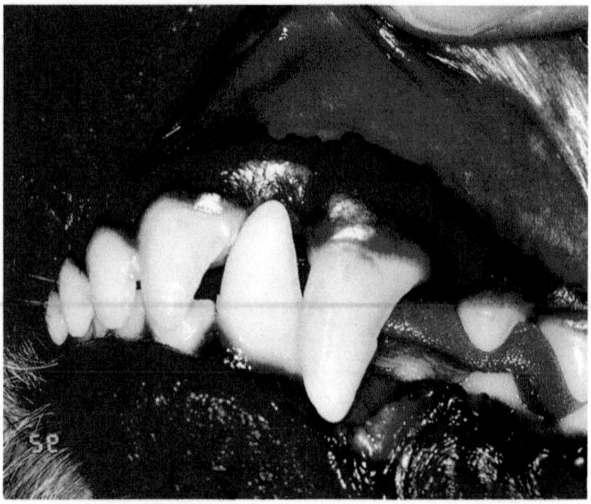

Fig. 5.2 Interdigitation of the canine teeth. There should be equal space on either side of the mandibular canine crown.

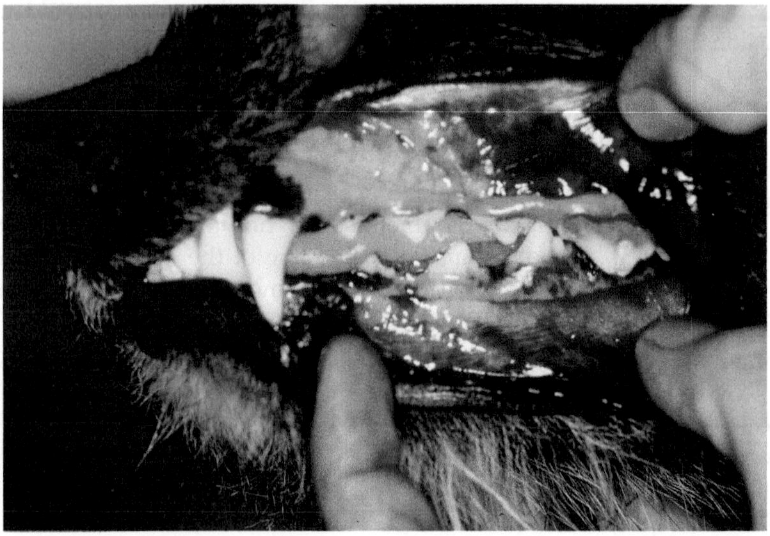

Fig. 5.3 Interdigitation of the premolars. This interdigitation is called the 'pinking shear' effect.

- The incisal tips of the mandibular incisors contact the cingulae of the upper incisors

Interdigitation of the canine teeth (Fig. 5.2)

- The mandibular canine fits into the diastema (space) between the upper 3rd incisor and the upper canine, touching neither. In other words, there should be equal space on either side of the mandibular canine crown

The incisor scissor bite and canine interdigitation form the dental interlock, which coordinates rostral growth of the upper jaw and mandible.

Interdigitation of the premolars (Fig. 5.3)

- The cusps (tips) of the premolars oppose the interdental spaces of the opposite arcade, with the mandibular 1st premolar being the

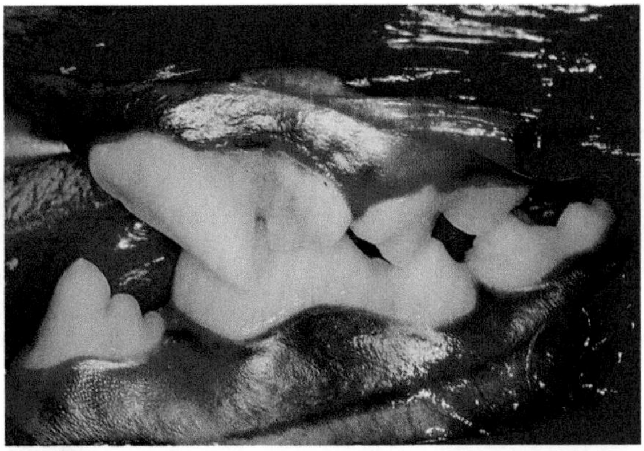

Fig. 5.4 Premolar and molar relationships in the dog. The mesiobuccal surface of the 1st mandibular molar occludes with the palatal surface of the maxillary 4th premolar and the distal occlusal surface of the mandibular 1st molar occludes with the palatal occlusal surface of the maxillary 1st molar.

most rostral. This interdigitation is called the 'pinking shear' effect

Premolar and molar relationships (Fig. 5.4)

- The mesiobuccal surface of the 1st mandibular molar occludes with the palatal surface of the maxillary 4th premolar
- The distal occlusal surface of the mandibular 1st molar occludes with the palatal occlusal surface of the maxillary 1st molar

Cat

The incisor and canine occlusion of the adult mesocephalic cat is the same as in the dog. The premolar and molar occlusion differs (Fig. 5.5) from the dog as follows:

- The most rostral premolar is the maxillary 2nd premolar (the cat lacks the 1st maxillary premolar and the first two mandibular premolars)
- The buccal surface of the 1st mandibular molar occludes with the palatal surface of the maxillary 4th premolar
- The maxillary 1st molar is located distopalatal to the maxillary 4th premolar and does not occlude with any other tooth

The cat does not have any teeth with occlusal (chewing) surfaces.

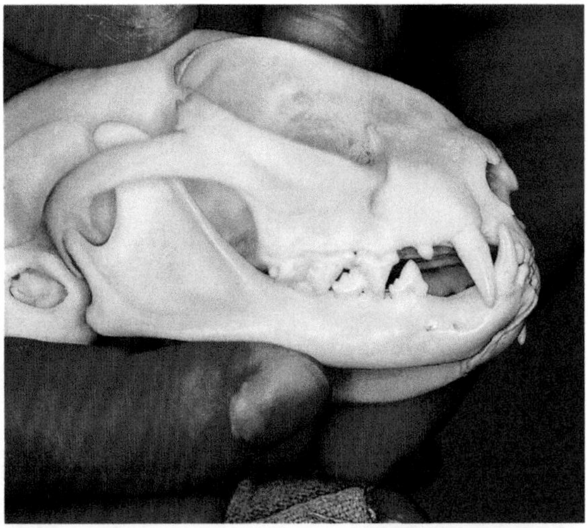

Fig. 5.5 Premolar and molar relationships in the cat. The most rostral premolar is the maxillary 2nd premolar. The buccal surface of the 1st mandibular molar occludes with the palatal surface of the maxillary 4th premolar. The maxillary 1st molar is located distopalatal to the maxillary 4th premolar and does not occlude with any other tooth.

SKELETAL MALOCCLUSION

Brachycephalic dogs have a shorter than normal upper jaw (Fig. 5.6) and dolicocephalic dogs have a longer than normal upper jaw (Fig. 5.7); in both cases the mandible is not responsible for any rostrocaudal discrepancy of the occlusion.

Mandibular prognathic bite

In the mandibular prognathic bite, often called 'undershot' (Fig. 5.8), the mandible is longer than the maxilla and some or all of the mandibular teeth are rostral to their normal position. The degree of malocclusion varies as follows:

- Normal incisor occlusion, but the mandibular canines touch the upper 3rd incisors and the mandibular premolars are rostrally displaced, which disrupts the 'pinking shear' effect
- Level bite: the upper and lower incisors meet at their incisal edges; the lower canines touch the upper 3rd incisors and the mandibular premolars are rostrally displaced

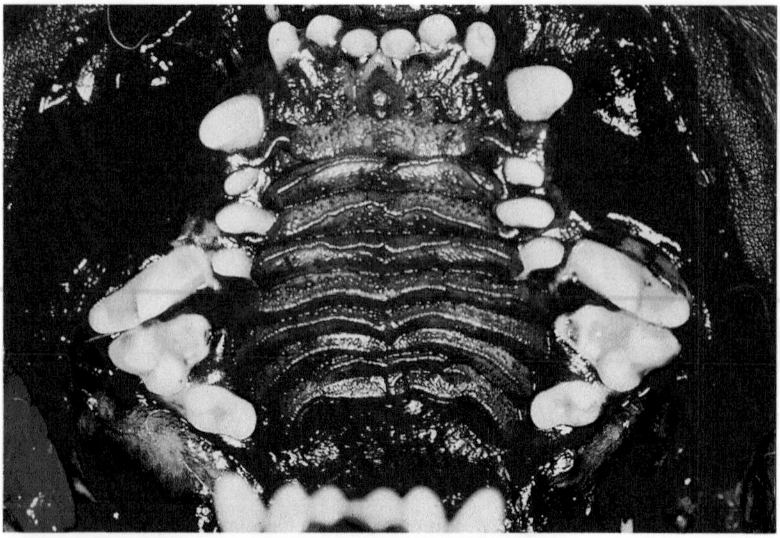

Fig. 5.6 Brachycephalic. Brachycephalic animals have a shorter than normal upper jaw. A short jaw results in reduced interdental spaces with rotation and/or overlap of teeth.

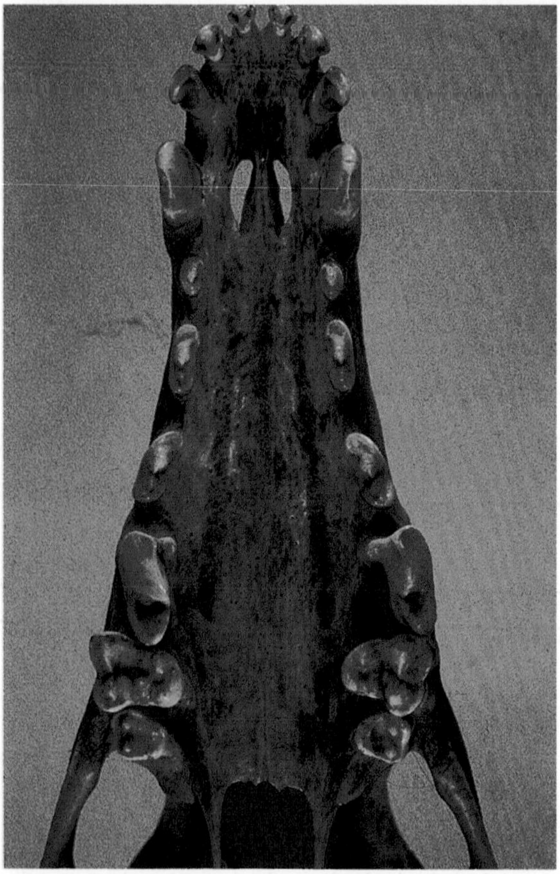

Fig. 5.7 Dolicocephalic. Dolicocephalic breeds have a longer than normal upper jaw. The increased jaw length results in interdental spaces that are wider than normal.

- Reverse scissor bite: the lower incisors are rostral to the upper incisors by 0.5 mm to 5 cm or more; the lower canines may be caudal to but touching the upper 3rd incisors, or may be rostral to the upper 3rd incisors; the mandibular premolars are rostrally displaced to a similar degree

If the dental interlock prevents the mandible from growing rostrally to its genetic potential, lateral or ventral bowing of the mandible may occur to accommodate the length. This results in an open bite and is characterised by increased space between the premolar cusp tips. In addition, the caudal angle of the mandible is caudal to the temporomandibular joint to accommodate the extra length of the mandible.

Mandibular brachygnathic bite

A mandibular brachygnathic bite, often called 'overshot', occurs when the mandible is shorter than normal (Fig. 5.9). The degree of malocclusion varies as follows:

- The upper incisors are rostral to the lower incisors by 0.5 mm to 5 cm or more
- The upper canines are caudal to but touching the mandibular canines; level with the lower canines; or rostral to the mandibular canines

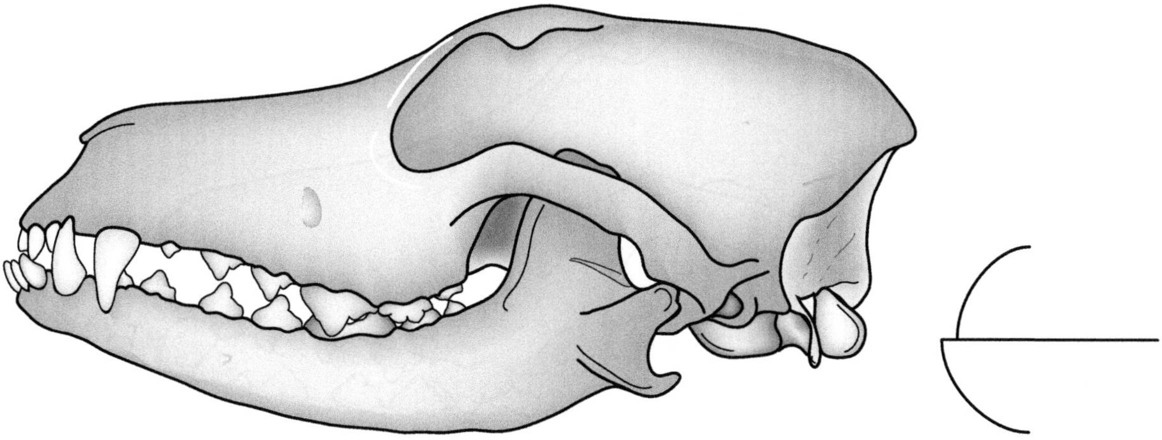

Fig. 5.8 Mandibular prognathic bite. The mandible is longer than the upper jaw.

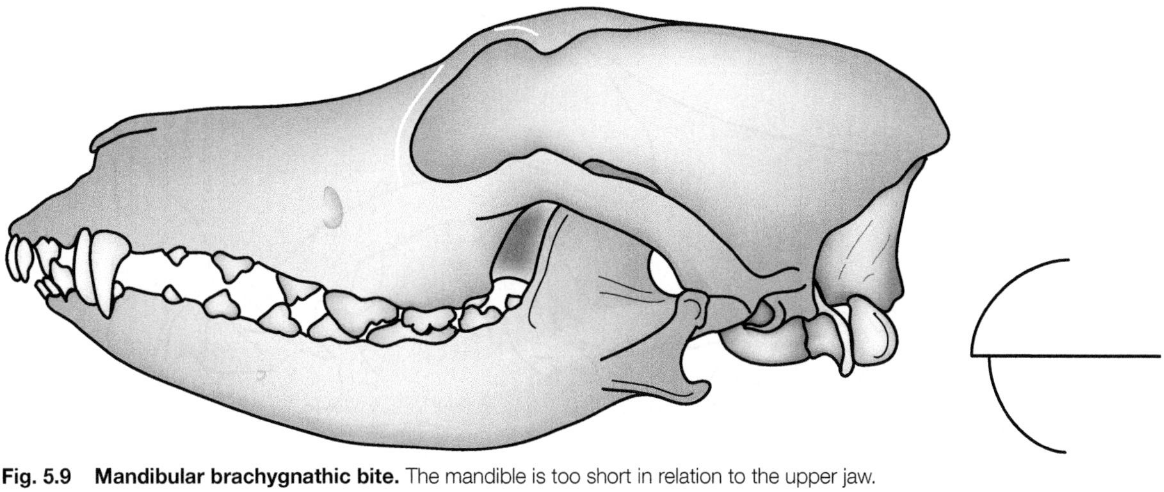

Fig. 5.9 Mandibular brachygnathic bite. The mandible is too short in relation to the upper jaw.

- The mandibular premolars are caudally displaced relative to the maxillary premolars, disrupting the 'pinking shear' effect. The degree of displacement is similar to that of the incisors and canines

Wry bite

A wry bite (Fig. 5.10) occurs if one side of the head grows more than the other side. In its mildest form a one-sided prognathic or brachygnathic bite develops. In more severe cases, a crooked head and bite develops with a deviated midline. An open bite may also develop in the incisor region so that the affected teeth are displaced vertically and do not occlude. The space between the upper and lower incisors can vary from 0.5 mm to 2 cm.

Narrow mandible

In some animals, the mandible is too narrow with respect to the upper jaw. The result is that the lower canines impinge on the maxillary gingivae

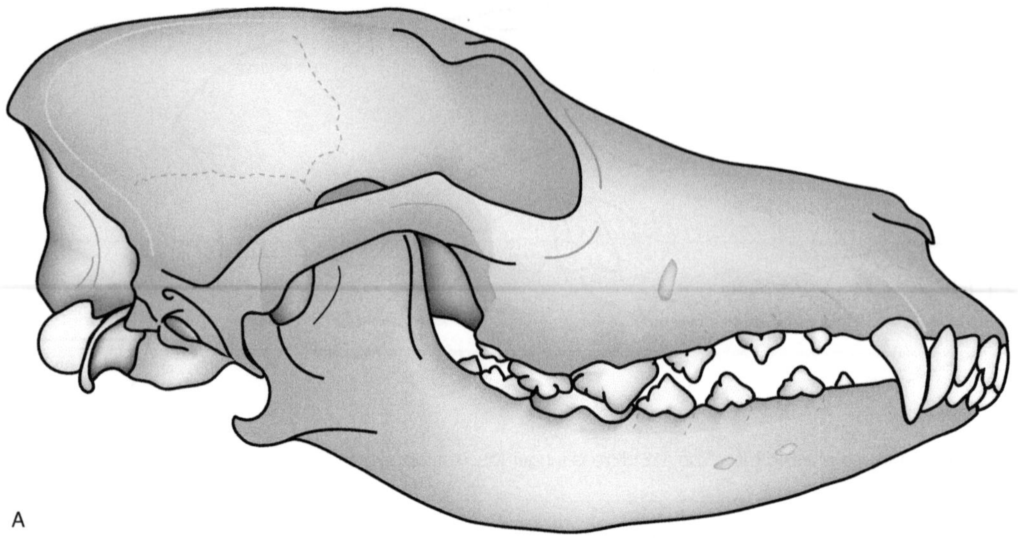
A

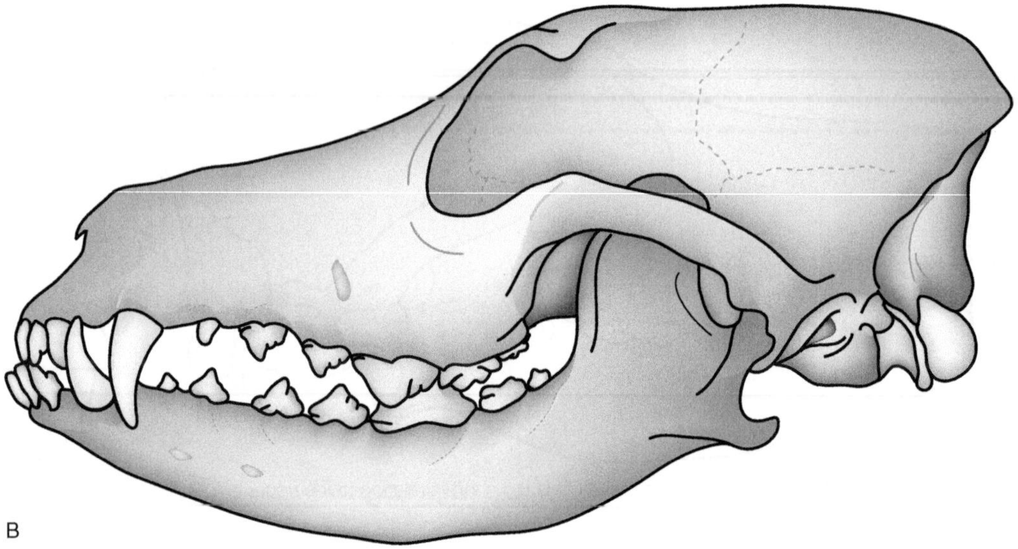
B

Fig. 5.10 Wry bite.
A: Right lateral view of the skull showing normal occlusion.
B: Left lateral view of the skull showing a mandibular prognathic bite.

or the hard palate instead of fitting into the diastema between the upper 3rd incisor and upper canine on either side (Fig. 5.11A, B). The animal may not be able to close its mouth and injury to the gingivae or palatal mucosa commonly occurs. In untreated severe cases, an oronasal communication may develop over time.

This condition is seen in both the primary (deciduous) and permanent dentition. Persistent primary canines will further exacerbate the condition as the permanent canines erupt medially to their primary counterparts in the mandible. The incorrect dental interlock will interfere with the normal growth in width and length of the developing mandible. The condition can also be caused by persistent primary mandibular canines in a mandible of normal width.

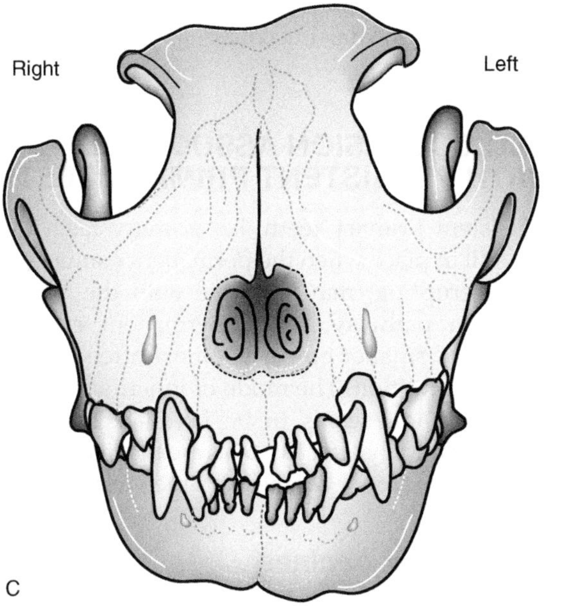

Fig. 5.10 Wry bite. *(contd)*
C: Rostral view of the skull showing a midline deviation and an open bite. Note that the left side of the skull is more developed than the right.

DENTAL MALOCCLUSION

Dental malocclusion is malpositioning of teeth where there is no obvious skeletal abnormality, i.e. there is no jaw length or width discrepancy. Dental malocclusion may also occur in association with skeletal malocclusion.

Anterior crossbite

This is a clinical term used to describe a reverse scissor occlusion of one, several or all of the incisors (Fig. 5.12). The condition is thought to be secondary to persistent primary incisors. However, there is probably a skeletal origin as well since affected animals often develop a mandibular prognathic bite. In other words, an anterior crossbite in an immature animal may be the first sign of a developing mandibular prognathism.

Anterior crossbite is common in medium and large breed dogs where persistent primary teeth are less common. The cause can be either a dental malocclusion (i.e. linguoversion of the upper incisors), or a skeletal malocclusion (i.e. mandibular prognathism or maxillary brachygnathism). Anterior crossbite in humans usually has a skeletal origin.

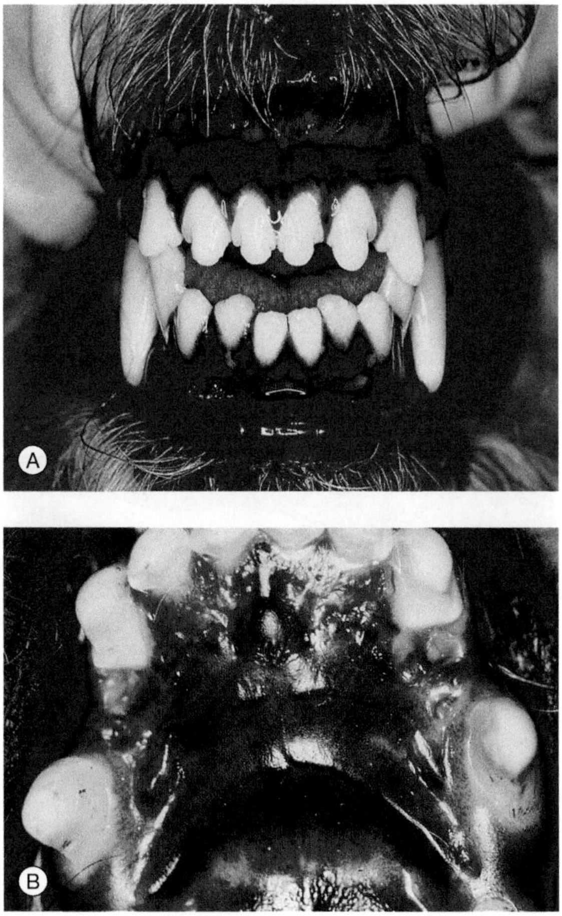

Fig. 5.11 Narrow mandible.
A: The mandibular canines do not fit into the diastema between the upper 3rd incisor and upper canine on either side. Instead, the mandibular canines impinge on the maxillary gingivae and hard palate. The dog is unable to close its mouth.
B: Note the injury to the maxillary gingivae and palatal mucosa.

Malocclusion of the canine teeth

The two most common abnormalities in canine tooth position are rostral displacement of the maxillary canines and medial displacement of the lower canines.

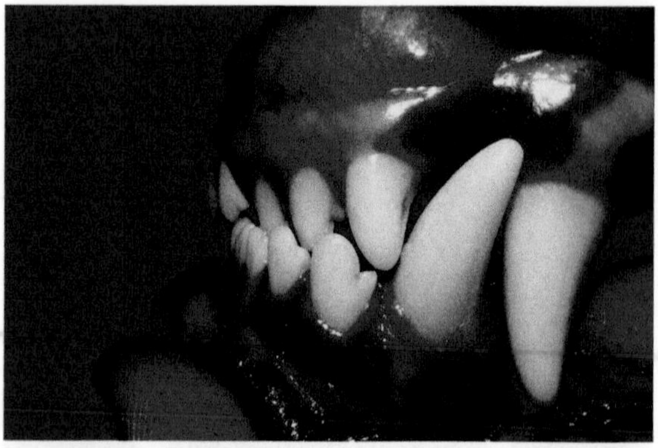

Fig. 5.12 Left anterior crossbite. The left incisors have a reverse scissor occlusion.

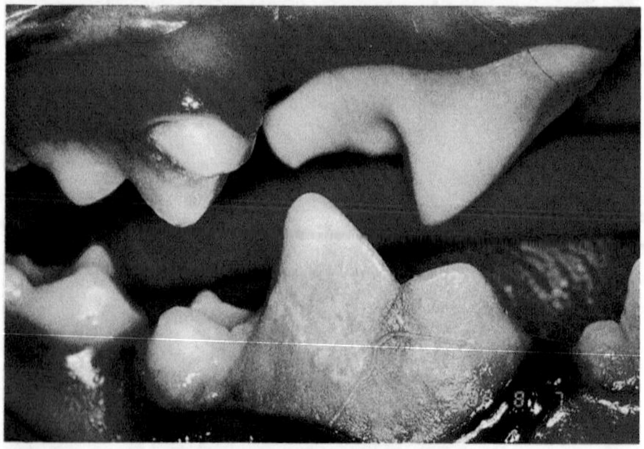

Fig. 5.13 Posterior crossbite. The normal buccolingual relationship of the carnassial teeth is reversed.

Rostral displacement of the maxillary canines

Persistent primary canines may be responsible for this condition. A breed predisposition has been reported in the Shetland sheepdog.

Medial displacement of the lower canines

Persistent primary mandibular canines are thought to be the cause of this condition. Yet, the condition is not frequent in toy breeds, where persistent primary teeth are common. This malocclusion is frequent in dolicocephalic breeds, where it is of skeletal origin in that the mandible is too small for the long maxilla.

Malocclusion of the premolars and molars

The term 'posterior crossbite' (Fig. 5.13) is used to describe an abnormal relationship of the carnassial teeth, seen commonly in the dolicocephalic breeds, where the normal buccolingual relationship is reversed.

MALOCCLUSION ASSOCIATED WITH PERSISTENT PRIMARY TEETH

Persistent primary teeth, i.e. primary teeth that are still in place when the permanent counterpart starts erupting, may interfere with the normal eruption pathway of the permanent counterparts. The smaller breeds are more often affected by this condition. The mode of inheritance is not known but it seems to be familial. The three most commonly affected areas are the mandibular canines, the upper canines and the incisors.

Mandibular canines

The mandibular permanent canine begins eruption medial to its primary counterpart. Once the primary tooth is lost, the permanent canine flares out laterally to occupy the diastema between the upper 3rd incisor and upper canine. If the primary canine is not lost, the permanent canine may be forced to continue erupting medial to the persistent primary counterpart and will impinge on the hard palate causing pain, inflammation and possibly, with time, an oronasal communication.

Maxillary canines

The maxillary permanent canine erupts rostral to its primary counterpart (Fig. 5.14). If the primary tooth is retained, this may force the permanent tooth to erupt into the diastema intended for the permanent mandibular canine. The following malocclusion situations could then develop:

- The maxillary or mandibular canine may become impacted, i.e. does not erupt fully
- The mandibular canine may push the upper 3rd incisor or the upper canine in a labial/buccal direction
- The mandibular canine may be forced to erupt medial to the maxillary canine, thus impinging on the hard palate with possible formation of an oronasal communication, if left untreated

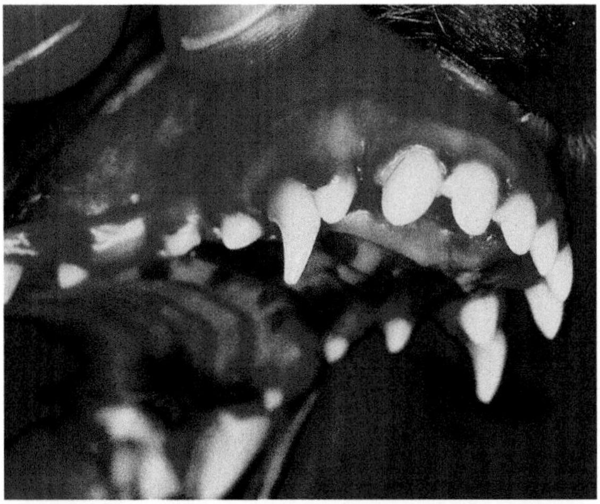

Fig. 5.14 Persistent primary maxillary canine. Due to the persistent primary maxillary canine, the permanent maxillary canine is being forced to erupt in the diastema that the permanent mandibular incisor normally occupies. Malocclusion will develop.

Incisors

The permanent incisors erupt caudal to their primary counterparts. Retention of one or more of the primary teeth may interfere with scissor occlusion of the permanent teeth, with upper incisors occluding behind the mandibular incisors, i.e. an anterior crossbite, which may result in localised soft tissue trauma.

DENTAL INTERLOCK-INDUCED ABNORMALITIES

A maloccluding dental interlock may form when a growth spurt of either the upper jaw or mandible coincides with the eruption of primary or permanent canines and incisors that interact to form the dental interlock. Once this interlock has been established the upper and lower jaws are forced to grow rostrally at the same rate, irrespective of the genetic information. For example, mandibular canines that are locked rostral to the upper 3rd incisors will cause a non-hereditary mandibular prognathic bite; mandibular canines that are locked medial and more caudal than normal will cause a narrow mandible and a mandibular brachygnathic bite.

PREVENTION AND TREATMENT OF MALOCCLUSION

Prevention is always better than treatment. Early recognition of a problem is essential to avoid discomfort and pain to the animal and prevent the development of severe pathology. Malocclusion affecting the primary dentition may require interceptive orthodontics. Malocclusion affecting the permanent dentition may need no treatment at all, if it is not causing the animal discomfort or any oral pathology. Malocclusion causing discomfort and pathology always needs treating.

Summary

- Malocclusion is common and may cause pain/discomfort and severe oral pathology
- It is essential to diagnose malocclusion early in the life of the animal
- Prevention is the best strategy
- Skeletal malocclusions and persistent primary teeth are hereditary
- In most instances, treatment, other than prevention, is best left to a veterinarian with special skills in dentistry
- The aim of any treatment is to make the animal comfortable with a functional bite; aesthetic considerations are of secondary importance

REFERENCES

Hennet, P.R. (1995) Orthodontics in small carnivores. In: Crossley, D.A. & Penman, S. (eds) *Manual of Small Animal Dentistry*. Cheltenham: BSAVA, pp. 182–192.

Hennet, P.R. & Harvey, C.E. (1992) Diagnostic approach to malocclusions in dogs. *Journal of Veterinary Dentistry* **9**(2): 23–26.

Stockard, C.R. (1941) The genetic and endocrinic basis for differences in form and behaviour. *The American Anatomical Memoirs No 19*. Philadelphia: The Wistar Institute of Anatomy and Biology.

6

Oral examination and recording

Examination of the oral cavity is part of every physical examination. Oral examination in a conscious animal will only give limited information. Definitive oral examination can only be performed under general anaesthesia. *All detected abnormalities should be recorded.* It saves time if one person performs the examination and another individual takes the notes and enters the findings on the dental record.

CONSCIOUS EXAMINATION

Oral examination of a conscious animal is limited to visual inspection and some digital palpation. Gentle technique is essential.

Examination involves not only assessing the oral cavity proper, but also palpation of:

- The face (facial bones and zygomatic arch)
- Temporomandibular joint
- Salivary glands (mandibular/sublingual; the parotids are usually only palpable if enlarged)
- Lymph nodes (mandibular, cervical chain)

Having looked at the entire face, the mouth is first examined by gently holding the jaws closed and retracting the lips (do not pull on the fur to retract lips) to look at the soft tissues and buccal aspects of the teeth. This is the optimal time to evaluate occlusion. Chapter 5 details the normal occlusal relationships in the dog and cat.

A checklist for evaluation of dental occlusion is shown in the box.

Six-point checklist for evaluation of dental occlusion

1. Head symmetry
2. Incisor relationship
3. Canine occlusion
4. Premolar alignment
5. Distal premolar/molar occlusion
6. Individual teeth positioning

After evaluating the occlusion, the animal is encouraged to open its mouth. One method of achieving this in the dog is to place a thumb and finger on the margin of the alveolar bone caudal to the canine teeth of the upper and lower jaw on one side and with gentle pressure encouraging the animal to open its jaws. Another method, useful for both dogs and cats, is to approach the animal from the side; one hand is placed over the muzzle and the lips are gently pressed into the oral cavity, while tilting the head slightly upwards. A finger from the other hand is placed on the lower incisors and gentle pressure is exerted. Do not use the fur under the mandible to try to pull the jaw down. Most animals allow at least a cursory inspection of the oral cavity once the jaws have been opened. The mucous membranes of the oral cavity should be examined as well as the teeth. Apart from colour and texture of the mucous membranes, look for evidence of a potential bleeding problem (petechiation, purpura, ecchymoses). In addition, look for vesicle formation, ulceration, which could indicate a vesiculobullous disorder, e.g. pemphigus, pemphigoid. Obvious pathology (tooth fracture, gingival recession, advanced furcation exposure) relating to the teeth can be identified. Assess the oropharynx (soft palate, palatoglossal arch, tonsillary crypts, tonsils and fauces) if possible. It is useful to identify any potential problems with endotracheal intubation prior to inducing anaesthesia.

EXAMINATION UNDER GENERAL ANAESTHESIA

The oropharynx should be examined prior to endotracheal intubation.

Normal anatomical features of the oral cavity need to be identified and inspected. Refreshing your memory on these features from an anatomy textbook is highly recommended. It is only with knowledge of the normal that abnormalities can be identified.

A series of useful checklists are shown in the box.

Checklists for oral examination under general anaesthesia

Oropharynx
- Soft palate
- Palatoglossal arch
- Tonsillary crypts
- Tonsils
- Hamular process of the pterygoid
- Fauces

Lips and cheeks
- Mucocutaneous junction
- Vestibules
- Philtrum
- Frenula (maxillary and mandibular)
- Salivary papilla (parotid and zygomatic)

Oral mucous membranes
- Alveolar mucosa
- Mucogingival line
- Attached gingiva
- Free gingiva

Hard palate
- Incisive papilla
- Incisive duct openings
- Palatine raphe and rugae

Floor of mouth and tongue
- Sublingual caruncle
- Lingual frenulum
- Lingual salivary gland (cat)
- Tongue papillae (types and distribution)

Teeth
- Primary, permanent or mixed dentition
- Missing and/or supernumerary teeth
- Abnormalities in size and/or shape
- Abnormalities in angulation and/or position
- Wear patterns (abrasion, attrition)
- Pathology, e.g. caries, enamel hypoplasia, tooth fracture

Periodontium

The periodontium of each tooth needs to be assessed. Examination of the periodontium is not routinely performed in veterinary practice. It is essential to perform a thorough periodontal examination in order to identify disease and plan treatment. The procedure for examination of the periodontium is detailed in the following.

Instruments required include:

1. Periodontal probe
2. Dental explorer
3. Dental mirror

The following indices and criteria should be evaluated for each tooth:

1. Gingivitis and gingival index
2. Periodontal probing depth
3. Gingival recession
4. Furcation involvement
5. Mobility
6. Periodontal (clinical) attachment level

In animals with large accumulations of dental deposits (plaque and calculus) on the teeth, it may be necessary to remove these to assess periodontal status accurately (Fig. 6.1A, B).

The purpose of the meticulous periodontal examination is to:

- Identify the presence of periodontal disease (gingivitis and periodontitis)
- Differentiate between gingivitis (inflammation of the gingiva) and periodontitis (inflammation

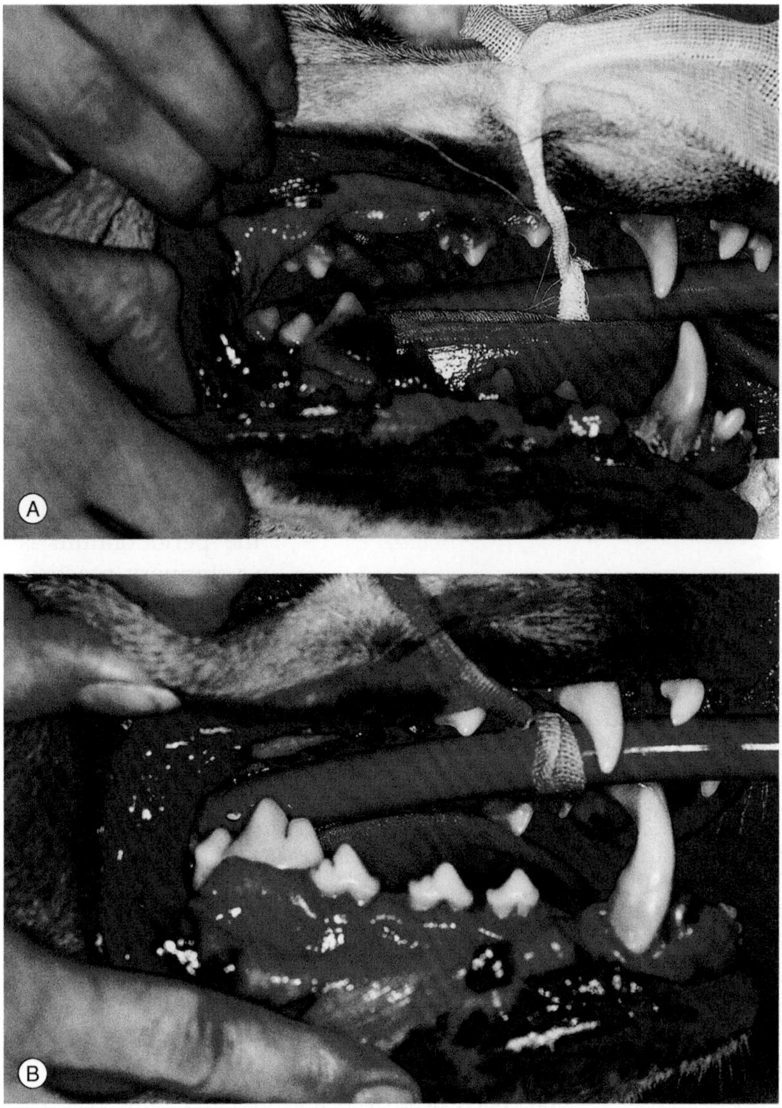

Fig. 6.1 Dental deposits and periodontal examination.
A: Large amounts of plaque and calculus make it impossible to assess the severity of periodontitis.
B: The periodontal destruction is evident once the dental deposits have been removed.

of the periodontal tissues resulting in loss of attachment and eventually tooth loss)
- Identify precise location of disease processes
- Assess the extent of tissue destruction where there is periodontitis

Periodontal probing depth, gingival recession, furcation involvement and mobility quantify the tissue destruction in periodontitis. Radiography to visualise the extent and type of alveolar bone destruction is mandatory if clinical evidence of periodontitis is found. Radiography of the jaws and teeth is detailed in Chapter 7. In many cases, measuring or calculating the periodontal or clinical attachment level (PAL/CAL) is also useful.

Gingivitis and gingival index

The presence and degree of gingivitis (inflammation of the gingiva) is assessed based on a combination of redness and swelling, as well as presence or absence of bleeding on gentle probing

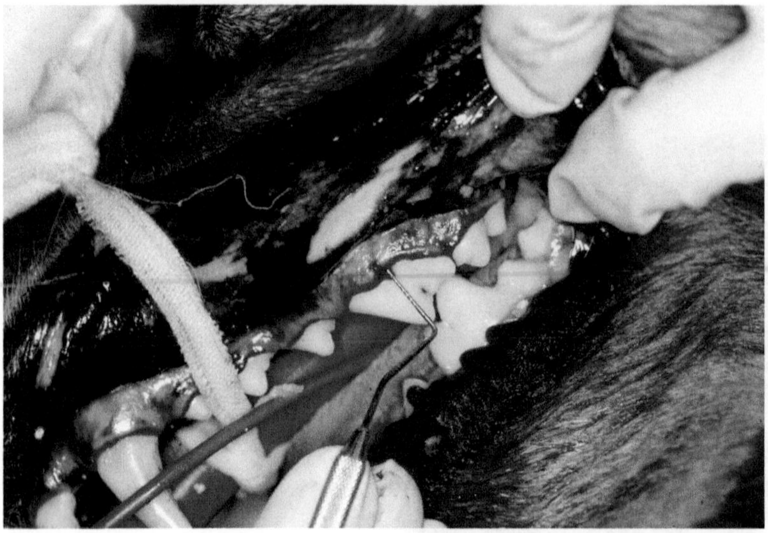

Fig. 6.2 Gingivitis scoring using the 'bleeding index'. A periodontal probe is gently inserted into the gingival sulcus at several locations around the whole circumference of each tooth; and given a score of 0 if there is no bleeding and a score of 1 if the probing elicits bleeding.

of the gingival sulcus. Various indices can be used to give a numerical value to the degree of gingival inflammation present. In the clinical situation, a simple bleeding index is the most useful. Using this method, a periodontal probe is gently inserted into the gingival sulcus at several locations around the whole circumference of each tooth; and given a score of 0 if there is no bleeding and a score of 1 if the probing elicits bleeding (Fig. 6.2).

An index which relies on both visual inspection and bleeding, namely the *modified* Löe and Silness gingival index (Löe, 1967), can also be used (Table 6.1). In research, this is the most commonly used method of assessing and quantifying gingivitis.

Table 6.1 The *modified* Löe and Silness gingival index

Gingival index 0	Clinically healthy gingiva
Gingival index 1	Mild gingivitis: slight reddening and swelling of the gingival margin; no bleeding on gentle probing of the gingival sulcus
Gingival index 2	Moderate gingivitis: the gingival margin is red and swollen; gentle probing of the gingival sulcus results in bleeding
Gingival index 3	Severe gingivitis: the gingival margin is red or bluish-red and very swollen; there is spontaneous haemorrhage and/or ulceration of the gingival margin

Periodontal probing depth (PPD)

The depth of the sulcus can be assessed by gently inserting a graduated periodontal probe until resistance is encountered at the base of the sulcus. The depth from the free gingival margin to the base of the sulcus is measured in millimetres at several locations around the whole circumference of the tooth (Fig. 6.3A, B). The probe is moved gently horizontally, walking along the floor of the sulcus. The gingival sulcus is 1–3 mm deep in the dog and 0.5–1 mm in the cat. Measurements in excess of these values usually indicate the presence of periodontitis when the periodontal ligament has been destroyed and alveolar bone resorbed, thus allowing the probe to be inserted to a greater depth. The term used to describe this situation is periodontal pocketing.

All sites with periodontal pocketing should be accurately recorded. Gingival inflammation resulting in swelling or hyperplasia of the free gingiva will, of course, also result in measuring sulcus depths in excess of normal values. In these situations, the term pseudopocketing is used, as the periodontal ligament and bone are intact (i.e. there is no evidence of periodontitis) and the increase in PPD is due to swelling or hyperplasia of the gingiva.

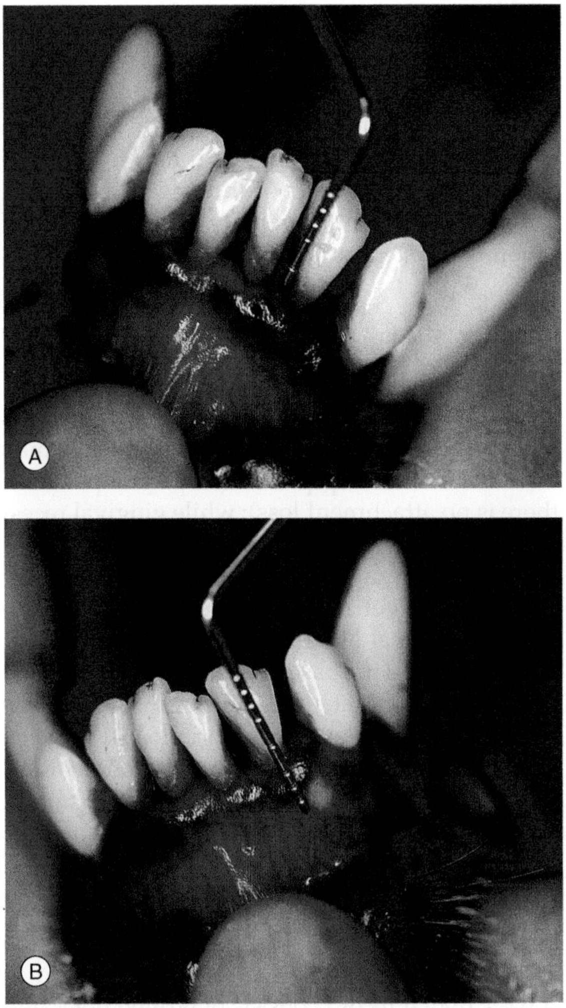

Fig. 6.3 Periodontal probing depth (PPD).
A: PPD is measured by inserting a periodontal probe into the gingival sulcus until firm resistance is felt. The distance from the free gingival margin to the depth of the sulcus or pocket is the periodontal probing depth. It should be measured and recorded at several sites around the circumference of each tooth. **B**: The probe has been placed on the surface of the gingiva to depict the depth to which it had been inserted.

Gingival recession

Gingival recession (Fig. 6.4) is also measured using a periodontal probe. It is the distance (in millimetres) from the cemento-enamel junction to the free gingival margin. At sites with gingival recession, PPD may be within normal values despite loss of alveolar bone due to periodontitis.

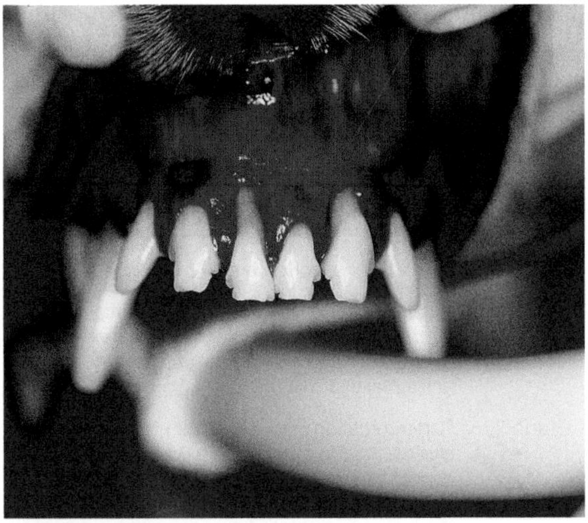

Fig. 6.4 Gingival recession. Gingival recession is measured from the cemento-enamel junction to the gingival margin using a graded periodontal probe. The right upper 1st incisor and the left upper 2nd incisor have an extensive (most of the root surface is exposed) gingival recession.

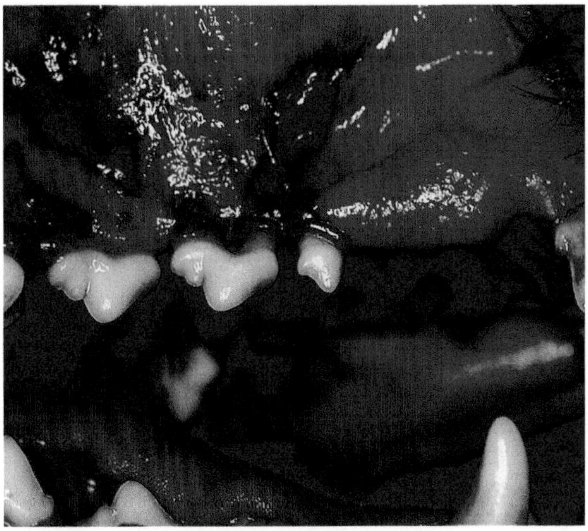

Fig. 6.5 Furcation involvement. The furcation sites of multirooted teeth should be examined with either a periodontal probe or a straight dental explorer so that the degree of furcation involvement can be graded. The right maxillary 2nd premolar has a grade 3 furcation, i.e. the explorer or probe can be passed through from buccal to palatal.

Furcation involvement

Furcation involvement refers to the situation where the bone between the roots of multirooted teeth is destroyed due to periodontitis (Fig. 6.5).

The furcation sites of multirooted teeth should be examined with either a periodontal probe or a straight dental explorer. The grading of furcation involvement is listed in Table 6.2.

Table 6.2 Grading of furcation involvement

Grade 0	No furcation involvement
Grade 1	Initial furcation involvement: the furcation can be felt with the probe/explorer, but horizontal tissue destruction is less than one-third of the horizontal width of the furcation
Grade 2	Partial furcation involvement: it is possible to explore the furcation but the probe/explorer cannot be passed through it from buccal to palatal/lingual. Horizontal tissue destruction is more than one-third of the horizontal width of the furcation
Grade 3	Total furcation involvement: the probe/explorer can be passed through the furcation from buccal to palatal/lingual

Table 6.3 Grading of tooth mobility

Grade 0	No mobility
Grade 1	Horizontal movement of 1 mm or less
Grade 2	Horizontal movement of more than 1 mm[a]
Grade 3	Vertical as well as horizontal movement is possible

[a] Note that multirooted teeth are scored more severely and a horizontal mobility in excess of 1 mm is usually considered to be grade 3 even in the absence of vertical movement.

Tooth mobility

The extent of tooth mobility should be assessed using a suitable instrument, e.g. the blunt end of the handle of a dental mirror or probe. It should not be assessed using fingers directly, since the yield of the soft tissues of the fingers will mask the extent of tooth mobility. The grading of mobility is listed in Table 6.3.

Periodontal/clinical attachment level (PAL/CAL)

Periodontal probing depth is not necessarily correlated with severity of attachment loss. As already mentioned, gingival hyperplasia may contribute to a deep pocket (or pseudopocket if there is no attachment loss); while gingival recession may result in the absence of a pocket but also minimal remaining attachment. Periodontal attachment level records the distance from the cemento-enamel junction (or from a fixed point on the tooth) to the base or apical extension of the pathological pocket. It is thus a more accurate assessment of tissue loss in periodontitis. PAL is either directly measured with a periodontal probe, or it is calculated (e.g. PPD + gingival recession).

RECORDING

The information resulting from the examination and any treatment performed needs to be recorded. A basic dental record consists of written notes and a completed dental chart. Additional diagnostic tests and radiographs are included as indicated.

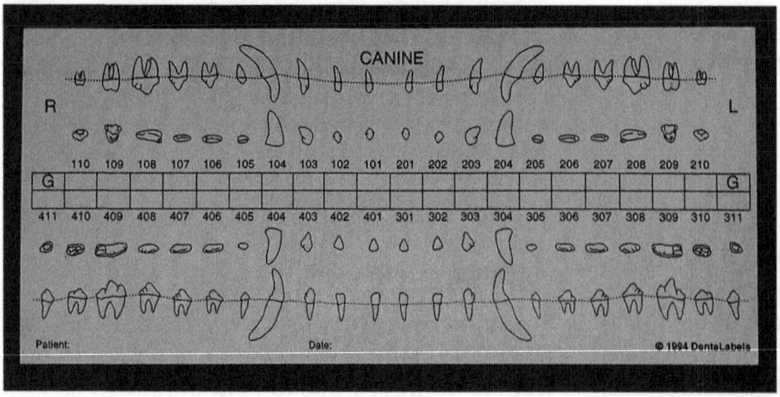

Fig. 6.6 Dentalabels®. A Dentalabel® (available for dog and cat) is a simple way of recording most of your findings and treatments. However, it is only a chart and needs to be supplemented by clinical notes, radiographs, etc. to make a complete dental record.

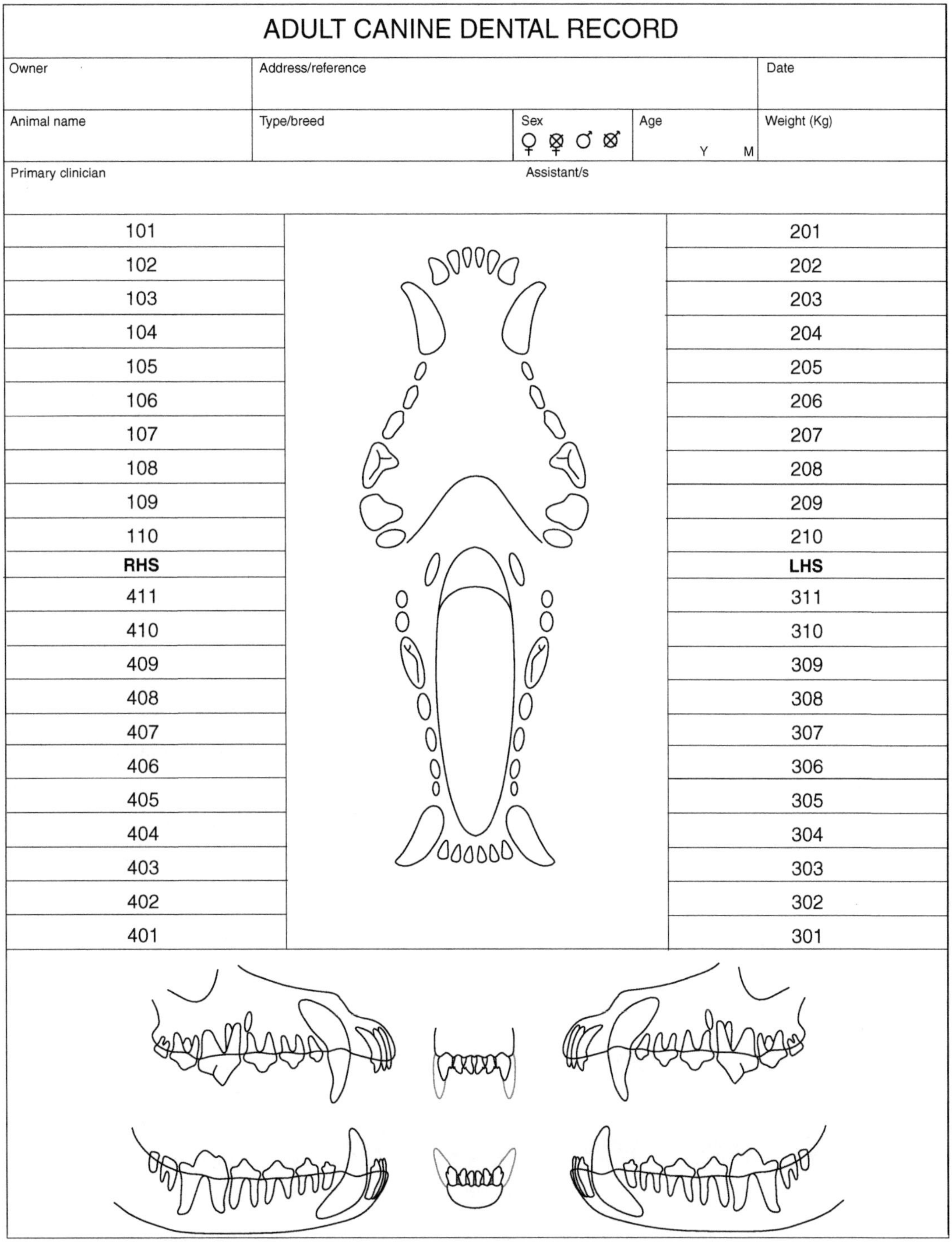
ADULT CANINE DENTAL RECORD

Owner	Address/reference			Date
Animal name	Type/breed	Sex ♀ ⊗ ♂ ⊗	Age Y M	Weight (Kg)
Primary clinician		Assistant/s		

RHS		LHS
101		201
102		202
103		203
104		204
105		205
106		206
107		207
108		208
109		209
110		210
RHS		**LHS**
411		311
410		310
409		309
408		308
407		307
406		306
405		305
404		304
403		303
402		302
401		301

Fig. 6.7 The EVDC dental record sheet. The basic dental record sheet recommended by the European Veterinary Dental College (EVDC) can also be used in a general practice situation. It allows space for clinical notes. Findings and treatment can be recorded using the diagnostic and treatment codes and abbreviations. (Reproduced with permission of the European Veterinary Dental College.)

Diagnostic codes & abbreviations			Treatment codes & abbreviations
nnn = tooth number (e.g.104) n = measurement in mm O = missing tooth # = fracture (tooth or bone) *line drawn on chart* + = severity + to +++ 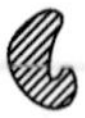 = location of lesion *drawn on chart*	A = abscess Ca = cavity (caries/resorption) C+ = calculus index (+ to +++) F+ = furcation (+ to +++) G+ = gingivitis (+ to +++) GH = gingival hyperplasia GR = gingival recession M+ = mobility (scale 1–3) ONF = oro-nasal fistula	ORL = resorptive lesion P = periodontal pocket Pn = probing depth (mm) Pi+ = plaque index (+ to +++) Rn = recession depth (mm) Snnn = supernumerary tooth St = staining (scale 1–3) U = ulcer	A = assessment T/Tx = therapy/treatment PT = periodontal therapy/treatment X = extraction/extracted S/Sx = surgery (e.g. SX/GSx) B = biopsy (e.g. SB/FNAB) E = endodontic (e.g. Epc/Erf/SxE) Epc = Tx vital pulp (capping) Erf = conventional root filling O = orthodontic (e.g. OA/OTx) R = restorative (e.g. R-composite)

Comments and further information

Adult

Skull type	Dolicocephalic	Normal	Brachycephalic
Jaw relationships	Mandibular prognathism	Normal	Mandibular brachy/retrognathism
Mandibular canine angulation		Normal	

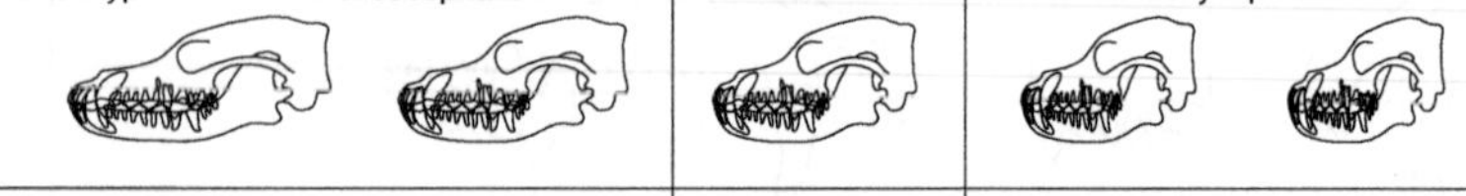

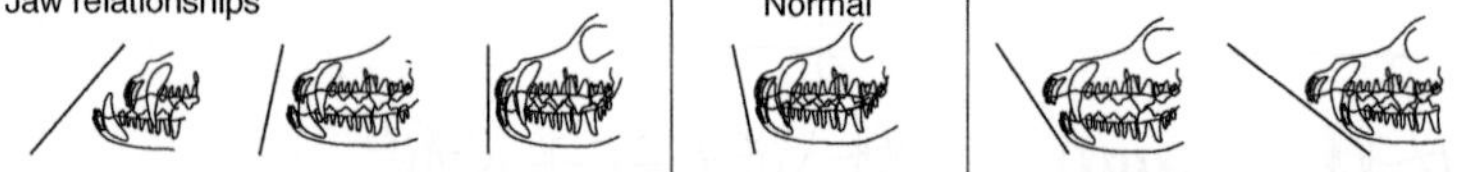

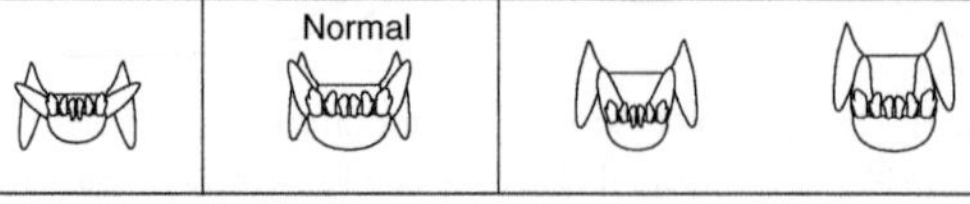

Case log entry number:		
A.	Oral medicine	
B.	Routine perio. Tx	
C.	Involved perio. Tx	
D.	Pocket reduction	
E.	Involved perio. Tx	
F.	Conventional endo. Tx	
G.	Vital pulp Tx	
H.	Surgical endodontics	
I.	Involved restoration	
J.	Crown and/or bridge	
K.	Simple extractions	
L.	Involved extractions	
M.	Jaw fracture fixation	
N.	Involved oral surgery	
O.	Other oral surgery	
P.	Orthodontic assessment	
Q.	Interceptive ortho. Tx	
R.	Simple orthodontic Tx	
S.	Involved orthodontic Tx	
T.	Other operative Tx	
U.	Non-cat/dog	
V.	In-vitro procedure	
W.	Primary responsibility	
X.	Imaging	
Y.	Other documentation	
Z.	Supervised by	

Fig. 6.7 The EVDC dental record sheet. *(contd)*

A completed dental record is a legal document that can be referred to:

- During treatment – to ensure that all treatment is performed
- At post-treatment discharge – to inform the owner of the condition of the teeth and of treatment performed
- At any time or by any person in the practice – for information related to the mouth at a specific date

A dental chart is a diagrammatic representation of the dentition, where information (findings and treatment) can be entered in a pictorial and/or notational form. A dental chart needs to be supplemented by clinical notes, radiographs, etc. to make a complete dental record. Dentalabel® (Fig. 6.6) is an example of a dental chart. It provides a simple way of recording most of your findings and treatments. In this chart, teeth are numbered using the modified Triadan system (Floyd, 1991), which is a three-digit numbering system. The first digit denotes the quadrant of the mouth and whether the tooth is part of the permanent or primary dentition, as shown in the box.

Permanent dentition	
Right upper = 1	Left upper = 2
Right lower = 4	Left lower = 3
Primary dentition	
Right upper = 5	Left upper = 6
Right lower = 8	Left lower = 7

The second and third digits together denote the tooth (see Fig. 6.6). In dogs the teeth are numbered consecutively from the rostral midline to the caudal end of each quadrant. In cats, where the complement of teeth is reduced (the 1st maxillary premolar and the 1st and 2nd mandibular premolars are absent, see Ch. 4), some numbers are skipped in the premolar region (West-Hyde, 1990).

The basic dental record sheet recommended by the European Veterinary Dental College (EVDC) can also be used in a general practice situation. They are currently available for the dog (puppy and adult) and the adult cat. The adult canine dental record is depicted in Figure 6.7. The EVDC dental records can be downloaded from the EVDC website (www.EVDC.info) free of charge.

The dental record recommended by the EVDC is continuously updated. It also contains information that is not relevant to the general practitioner, e.g. case log entry numbers, plaque and calculus index for all teeth, staining scale for all teeth. Our recommendation is to use the EVDC recommended record sheet as an example and draw up a dental record sheet suitable for the individual practice.

The dog and cat dental record sheets that we use are depicted in Figure 6.8A, B. The front is used to record clinical findings and the back is used to enter diagnosis, draw up a treatment plan and record treatment performed. The nurse or technician who performs the clinical examination completes the front page. The veterinarian checks the clinical findings and interprets any radiographs taken and then fills in the back page of the chart. Figure 6.8A depicts a blank record sheet and Figure 6.8B shows a completed form. Abbreviations are used when filling in the record sheet. It is important that a list of what the abbreviations mean is available. A list of commonly used abbreviations is found in Table 6.4.

Table 6.4 Common abbreviations

NAD	No abnormality detected
FORL	Feline odontoclastic resorptive lesion
GR	Gingival recession
GH	Gingival hyperplasia
UCF	Uncomplicated crown fracture
CCF	Complicated crown fracture
UCRF	Uncomplicated crown and root fracture
CCRF	Complicated crown and root fracture
W	Wear (abrasion or attrition) facet

Ⓐ

Dr Cecilia Gorrel BSc, MA, Vet MB, DDS, Hon FAVD, Dipl EVDC, MRCVS
Veterinary Dentistry and Oral Surgery Referrals, Veterinary Oral Health Consultancy

Client: ____________________
Animal: ____________________
Comp no: ____________________

DENTAL RECORD: DOG

Date: ____________________
Clinician: ____________________
Student: ____________________

OCCLUSAL EVALUATION	EXTRAORAL FINDINGS	ORAL SOFT TISSUES	OTHER RELEVANT FEATURES
Incisor occlusion: ______	______	______	______
Canine occlusion: ______	______	______	______
Premolar alignment: ______	______	______	______
Distal P/M occlusion: ______	______	______	______
Head symmetry: ______	______	______	______
Individual teeth: ______	______	______	______
Other: ______	______	______	______

PLAQUE

R/PM	R/IC	L/IC	L/PM

CALCULUS

R/PM	R/IC	L/IC	L/PM

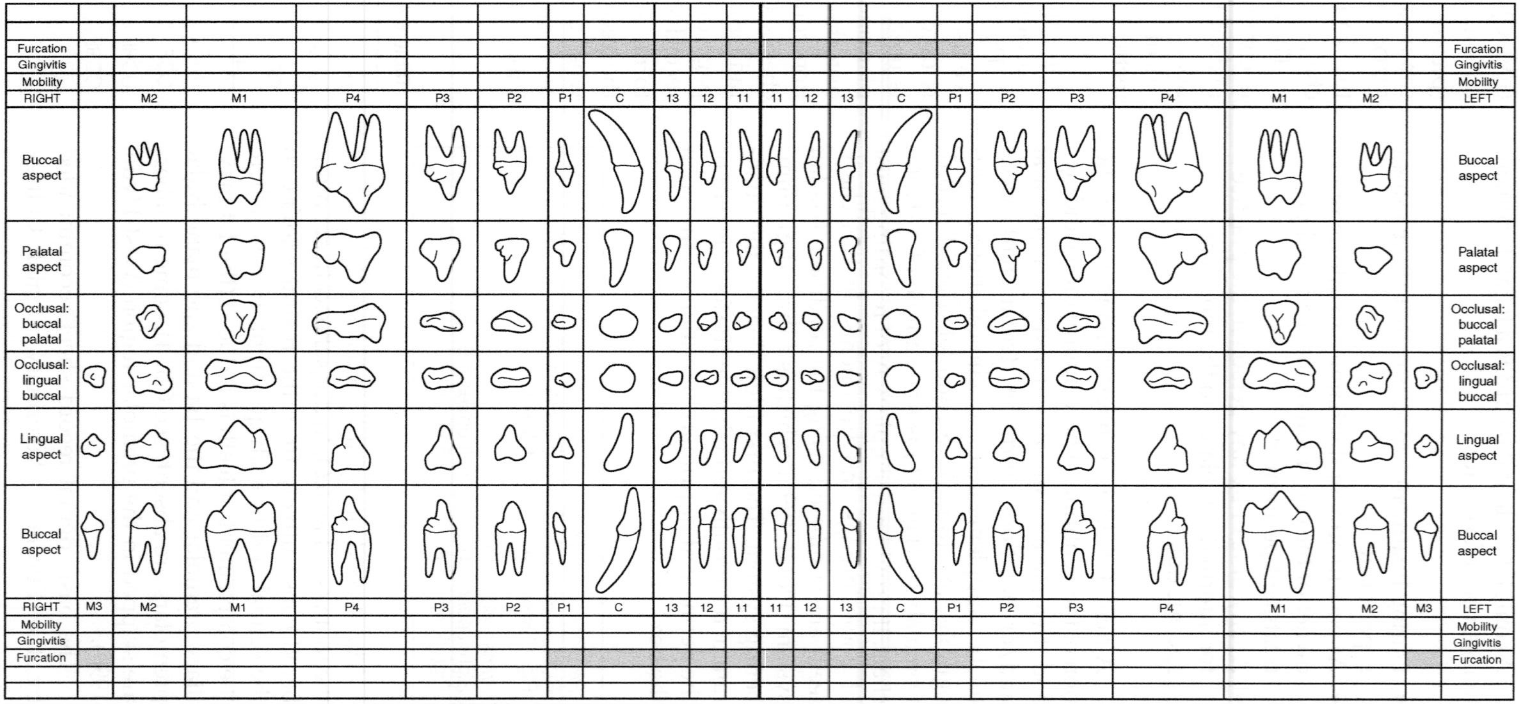

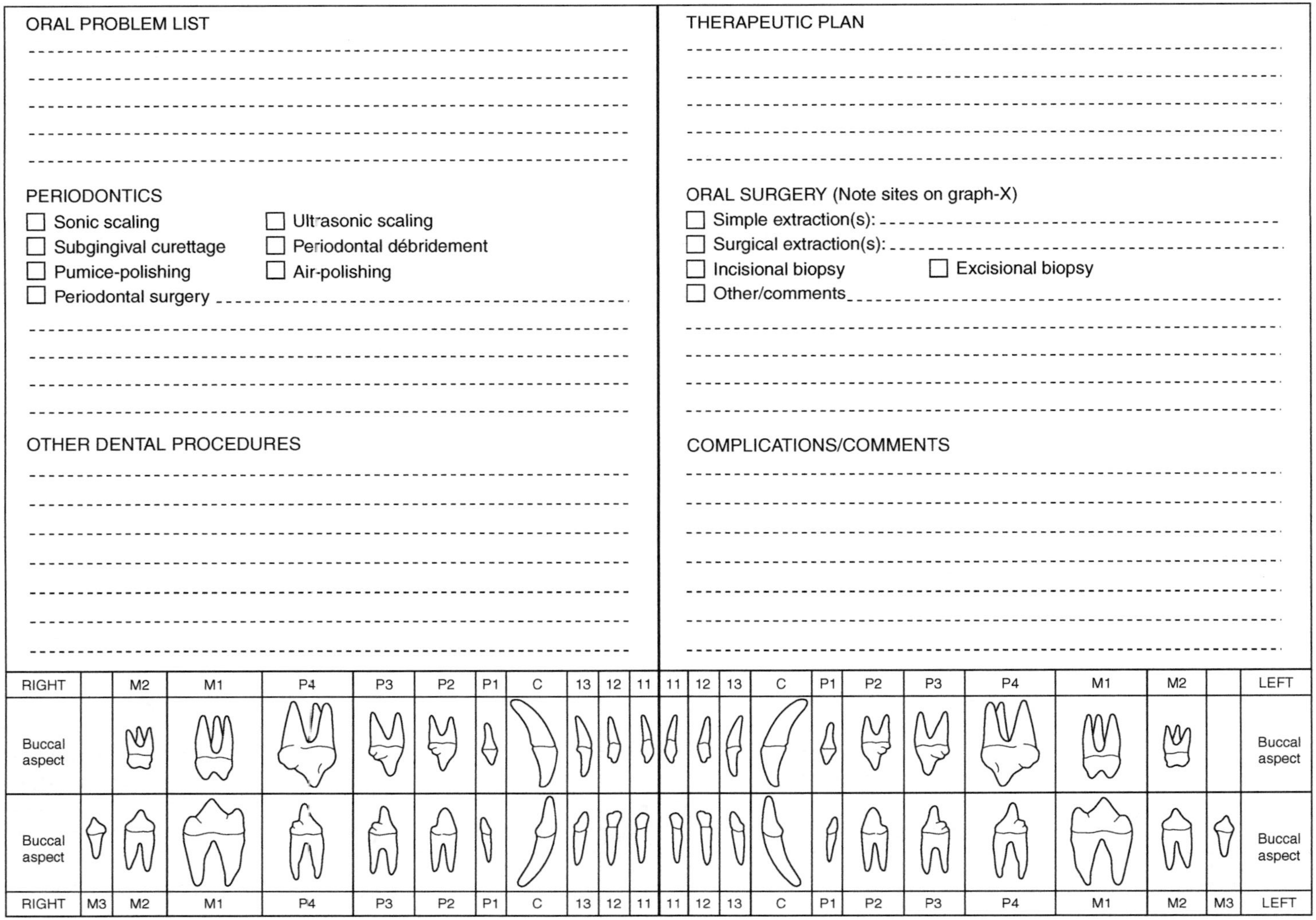
ORAL PROBLEM LIST

PERIODONTICS
☐ Sonic scaling
☐ Subgingival curettage
☐ Pumice-polishing
☐ Periodontal surgery
☐ Ultrasonic scaling
☐ Periodontal débridement
☐ Air-polishing

OTHER DENTAL PROCEDURES

THERAPEUTIC PLAN

ORAL SURGERY (Note sites on graph-X)
☐ Simple extraction(s):
☐ Surgical extraction(s):
☐ Incisional biopsy ☐ Excisional biopsy
☐ Other/comments

COMPLICATIONS/COMMENTS

RIGHT		M2	M1	P4	P3	P2	P1	C	13	12	11	11	12	13	C	P1	P2	P3	P4	M1	M2		LEFT
Buccal aspect																							Buccal aspect
Buccal aspect																							Buccal aspect
RIGHT	M3	M2	M1	P4	P3	P2	P1	C	13	12	11	11	12	13	C	P1	P2	P3	P4	M1	M2	M3	LEFT

Fig. 6.8 Our dental record sheets.
A: Blank dog dental record sheet. The front is used to record clinical findings and the back to note diagnoses, treatment plan and treatments performed.

(B)

Dr Cecilia Gorrel BSc, MA, Vet MB, DDS, Hon FAVD, Dipl EVDC, MRCVS
Veterinary Dentistry and Oral Surgery Referrals, Veterinary Oral Health Consultancy

DENTAL RECORD: CAT

Client: ________
Animal: ________
Comp no: ________

Date: ________
Clinician: ________
Student: ________
Nurse/Technician: ________

OCCLUSAL EVALUATION		EXTRAORAL FINDINGS	ORAL SOFT TISSUES	OTHER RELEVANT FEATURES
Incisor occlusion:	Normal occlusion			
Canine occlusion:		NAD	NAD	None
Premolar alignment:				
Distal P/M occlusion:				
Head symmetry:				
Individual teeth:				
Other:				

PLAQUE

R/PM	R/IC	L/IC	L/PM

CALCULUS

R/PM	R/IC	L/IC	L/PM

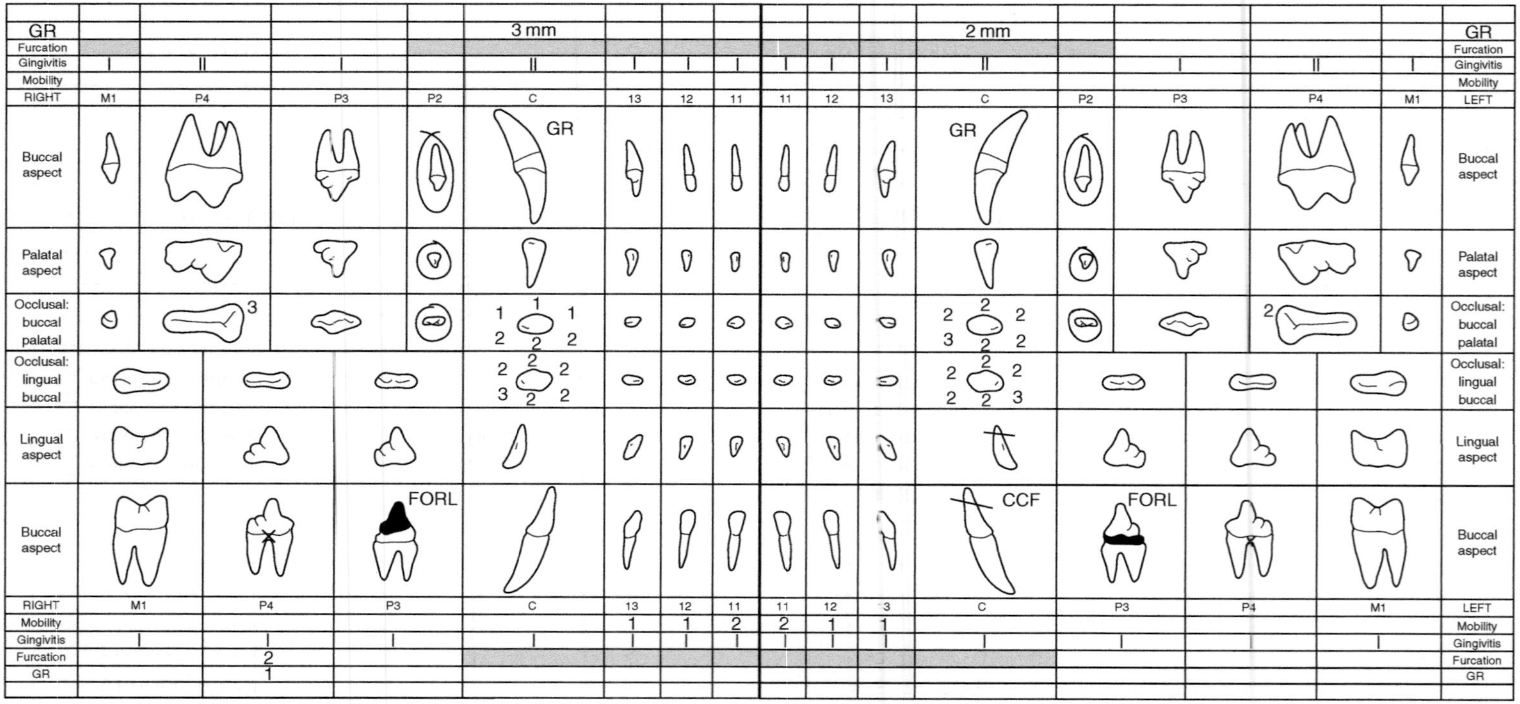

ORAL PROBLEM LIST

1) FORL 307, 407

2) CCF 304

3) Periodontitis 104, 204

4) 106 and 206 are missing

5) Mild generalised gingivitis

THERAPEUTIC PLAN (after reviewing radiographs)

1) Periodontal therapy

2) Extract 304, 307, 407

PERIODONTICS

- ☐ Sonic scaling
- ☑ Subgingival curettage
- ☑ Pumice-polishing
- ☐ Periodontal surgery
- ☑ Ultrasonic scaling
- ☐ Periodontal débridement
- ☐ Air polishing

ORAL SURGERY (Note sites on graph-X)

- ☐ Simple extraction(s):
- ☑ Surgical extraction(s):
- ☐ Incisional biopsy
- ☐ Excisional biopsy
- ☐ Other comments

OTHER DENTAL PROCEDURES

Full mouth radiographic series taken.

COMPLICATIONS/COMMENTS

Needs recall for EUA and full mouth radiographs in one year's time.

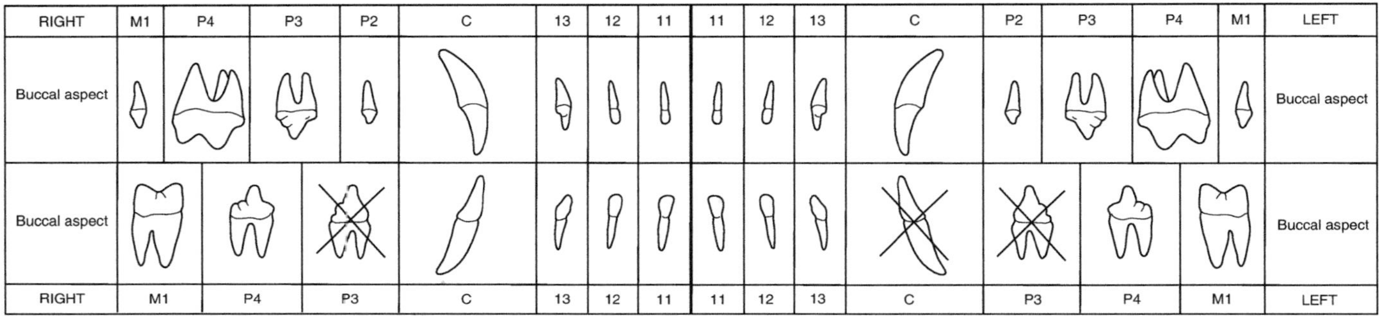

Fig. 6.8 Our dental record sheets. *(contd)*

B: Completed cat dental record sheet.

Plaque and calculus accumulation can be noted as mild, moderate or severe. We do not routinely score the degree of accumulation of plaque or calculus, as they will be removed during the periodontal therapy. Note that only abnormalities are recorded on the chart. Gingivitis has been recorded using the modified Löe and Silness gingival index. Sites with increased periodontal probing depths are marked on the occlusal view.

Summary

- Full oral examination is only possible under general anaesthesia
- Oral examination should proceed in an orderly and structured fashion, using appropriate instrumentation
- Several indices and measurements should be taken to complement visual assessments, e.g. gingival index, periodontal probing depth, gingival recession, furcation
- Adequate recording (of all findings) should take place
- A basic dental record consists of written notes and a dental chart. All findings and treatment should be marked here. This record should also be supplemented with radiographs etc

REFERENCES

Floyd, M.R. (1991) The modified Triadan System: Nomenclature for veterinary dentistry. *Journal of Veterinary Dentistry* **8**(4): 18–19.

Löe, H. (1967) The gingival index, the plaque index and the retention index system. *Journal of Periodontology* **38**: 610–616.

West-Hyde, L. (1990) The enigma of feline dentition. *Journal of Veterinary Dentistry* **7**(3): 16–17.

FURTHER READING

Gorrel, C. (1998) Radiographic evaluation. In: Holmstrom, S. (ed) *Canine Dentistry. Veterinary Clinics of North America: Small Animal Practice*. Philadelphia: WB Saunders, pp. 1089–1110.

Robinson, J. & Gorrel, C. (1995) Oral examination and radiography. In: Crossley, D.A. & Penman, S. (eds) *Manual of Small Animal Dentistry*. Cheltenham: BSAVA, Ch. 5, pp. 25–49.

7

Dental radiography

Radiography is a vital tool in veterinary dentistry. The bulk of the tooth, i.e. root and most of the periodontium, can only be visualised by means of radiographs. Consequently, a lot of pathology will remain undiscovered if clinical examination does not involve radiography. While lesions such as caries can be recognised without radiography it is not possible to assess the full extent of the lesions or if there is pulpal and periapical involvement. In other words, a clinical examination is incomplete without radiography. Periodontal disease, endodontic disease, caries, resorptive lesions, fractures, bone pathology and neoplastic conditions all require radiography for a more complete diagnosis, thus allowing optimal planning of treatment. Practising dentistry without taking radiographs would be considered negligent in human dentistry. The same applies to veterinary dentistry.

Pathological radiographic changes are usually discrete and therefore clarity and detail are essential. For a dental radiograph to be diagnostic, it should be an accurate representation of the size and shape of the tooth without superimposition of adjacent structures (Figs 7.1 and 7.2). Intraoral radiographic techniques are therefore required; a

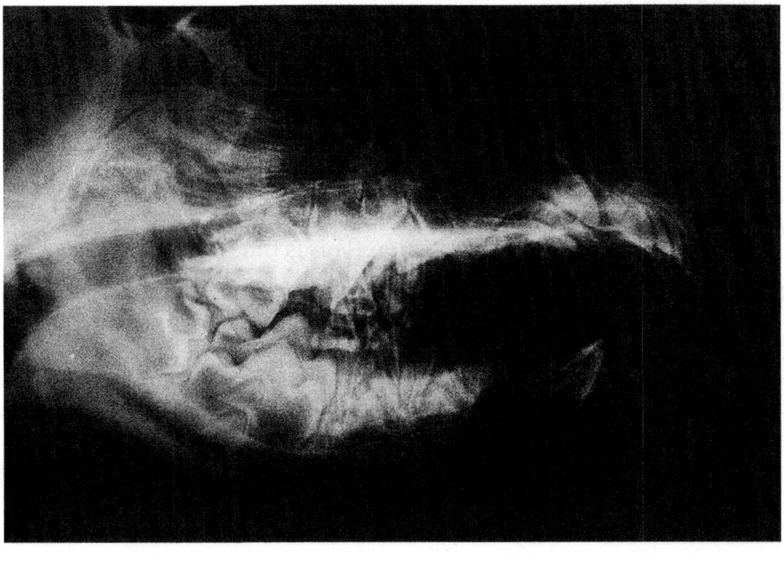

Fig. 7.1 A non-diagnostic view. This lateral view (extraoral film positioning) is non-diagnostic for evaluation of teeth and associated tissues. There is superimposition of the right and left side. In fact, it is not possible to say much more than that it is a radiograph of an immature dog and there are teeth present.

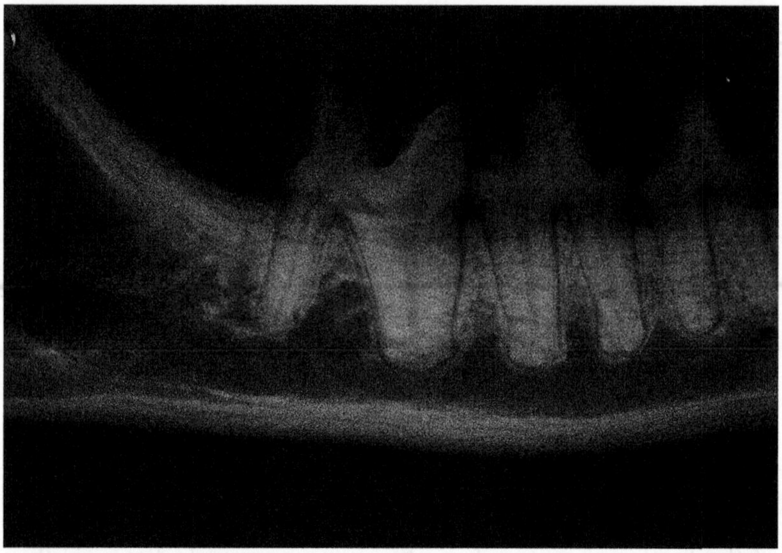

Fig. 7.2 A diagnostic view. For a dental radiograph to be diagnostic, it should be an accurate representation of the size and shape of the tooth without superimposition of adjacent structures.

Intraoral placement of dental film and parallel technique gives an accurate representation of the mandibular 3rd and 4th premolars and the 1st molar, as well as detail of the mandibular bone in this cat. The mesial surface of the 3rd premolar is not on the film and a second view with the film placed further rostrally in the mouth is required to assess this tooth fully.

In this view, the component structures of the tooth and its supporting tissues are well defined. The enamel is seen as an incompletely visualised radiodense band that covers the crown and tapers to a fine edge at the cervical margin of the tooth. The dentine is less radiodense than enamel and accounts for the bulk of the hard tissues of the tooth. Cementum is not visible radiographically. The pulp cavity is the continuous radiolucent space in the centre of the tooth that extends from the crown to the apex of the roots. The bony wall of the tooth socket (the lamina dura) is the radiodense line, which runs parallel to the root of the tooth. The periodontal ligament space is the fine radiolucent line between the lamina dura and the root of the tooth. The cortical bone on the crest of the alveolar ridge is continuous with the lamina dura. The mandibular canal is clearly visible.

parallel technique for the mandibular premolars and molars, and a bisecting angle technique for all other teeth. Contralateral (same teeth, opposite side) views should be taken as routine.

Intraoral radiographic techniques do require some time and patience to master, but once this has been achieved they provide valuable information. Attending a practical course to learn these techniques is strongly recommended.

EQUIPMENT AND MATERIALS

Equipment and materials for intraoral radiography

- X-ray machine
- X-ray film
- Processing facilities
- Mounts for film storage

The X-ray unit

Most veterinary X-ray machines can be used for dental radiography, but the film–focus distance will need to be adjusted to between 30–50 cm. The more manoeuvrable the head (in angulation and positioning) the better it is for intraoral techniques. With the less manoeuvrable units it is necessary to position the animal differently for each area requiring investigation. This is time-consuming.

A dental X-ray machine is preferable to a veterinary X-ray machine. The dental unit has a freely manoeuvrable head that allows accurate positioning with minimal adjustment in patient position. The cone of the dental unit will collimate the beam and provide the optimal film–focus distance.

Ideally a dental X-ray machine should be installed in the designated dental theatre (Fig. 7.3). They are available as wall-mounted or

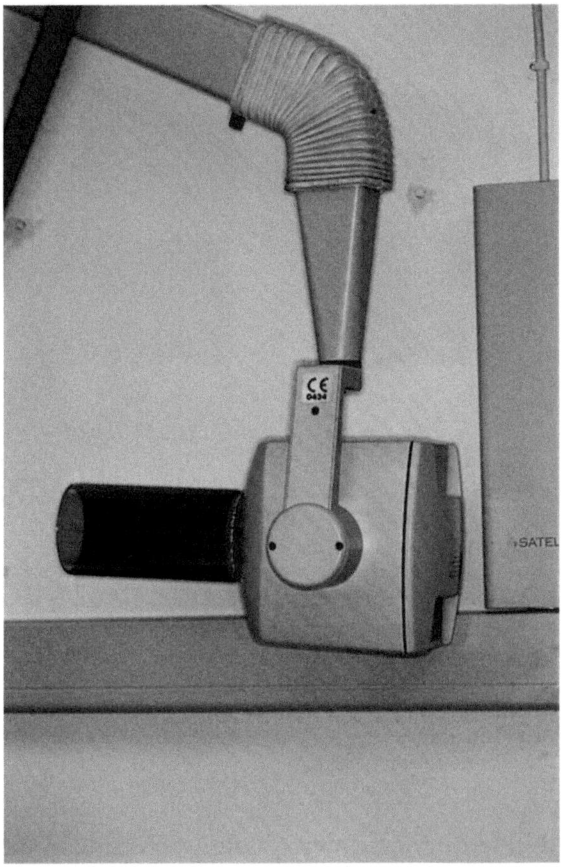

Fig. 7.3 A dental X-ray unit. A dental X-ray unit installed in the designated dental theatre is the ideal situation. These units are available as free-standing or wall-mounted. Wall-mounting is usually preferable to save space.

free-standing units. These machines are cost effective and their outlay is rapidly recouped. They usually have a fixed kV of 50–70 and a fixed mA of 8–10. Electronic timers are used to set the desired exposure time.

X-ray film

Single emulsion, non-screen or screen film can be used to take dental radiographs. To allow intra-oral film placement and achieve high definition, dental film should be used. Dental film is single emulsion, non-screen, and is available in three sizes (Fig. 7.4): occlusal, periapical and paediatric. It is available in two speeds: D (ultra) and E (Ekta). Ekta film has larger crystals in the film emulsion and is therefore faster. However, the resolution is poorer. The advantage of using the latter is that the film requires a lower exposure; however, E speed film cannot be developed in a chair-side developer. The dental film is packed in either a paper or a plastic envelope and the film is flanked by black paper and backed by a thin lead sheet (foil) that reduces scattered radiation.

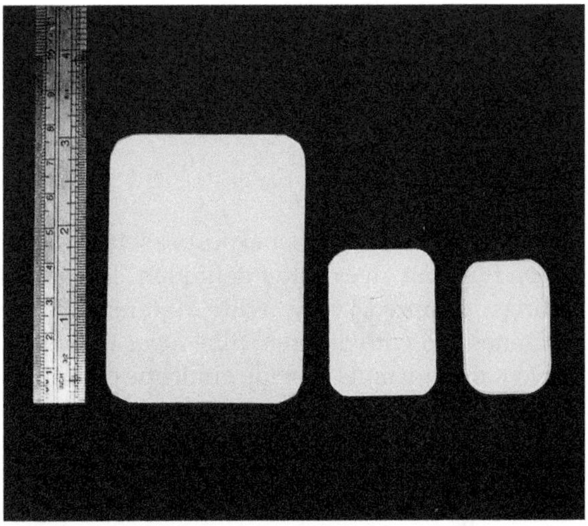

Fig. 7.4 Sizes of dental film. Dental film is available in three sizes, namely occlusal (5 × 7 cm), periapical (3 × 4 cm) and paediatric (2 × 3 cm). The smallest film that depicts the area of interest should be used to facilitate film positioning in the mouth.

Orientation

Ensure the correct side of the film envelope is facing the incident beam; the envelope is marked or labelled. If exposed through the back of the envelope, the lead sheet will absorb much of the X-ray beam, resulting in an underexposed radiograph with the pattern of the lead sheet imposed on it.

Each film has a raised dot in one corner. The dot helps with orientation when viewing and mounting dental radiographs if the following procedure is adhered to. First, the dot should face the incident beam. Secondly, the film should be placed in the mouth so that the dot is always facing a specific direction. We position the dot so that it is always facing forward in the mouth. Another way of doing it is to ensure that the film is placed so that the dot is always in the same position, i.e. facing forward in the mouth on one side and backward in the mouth on the contralateral side.

Exposure settings

Dental film requires higher exposure settings than screen film, but gives better definition. The actual settings required vary with different X-ray machines and with different film–focus distances.

Dental X-ray units provide guideline exposures for different size patients and different teeth. The X-ray unit is brought as close to the tooth that is being radiographed as possible, so setting film–focus distance is not required.

If you are using a veterinary X-ray unit and D speed dental film, set the film–focus distance between 30 and 50 cm and try the exposures suggested in the box.

Suggested exposure settings

Cat/small dog	60–70 kV	20–25 mA
Medium/large dog	70–80 kV	20–25 mA
Rabbit/guinea pig	50–60 kV	10–20 mA
Chinchilla	50–60 kV	5–15 mA

Irrespective of the type of X-ray unit available, it is advisable to take series of trial exposures on animals of different size to make up exposure charts prior to undertaking dental radiography on patients.

Dental film processing

Automated processors are available for dental film processing, but excellent results can be obtained with the use of a chair-side processor (Fig. 7.5). These chair-side 'darkrooms' have four containers, one each for developing and fixing fluids and two for rinsing purposes. Care must be exercised during processing to prevent scratching of the film surface. The films are held in the clip and passed through developer, rinse (water), fixer, and rinse (water). Development and fixation (gently agitating the film in the solutions), depending on manufacturer, is usually 30 seconds in each. Films must be adequately fixed so as not to lose quality during archiving. After processing in the Rinn box, thorough rinsing under running water, while gently rubbing the film surface with your fingers (not just agitating the film in the final rinse cup), is essential to avoid fixation stains. Rinsing is complete when the film surface no longer feels 'soapy'. Remember that E speed film should not be processed using a chair-side processor.

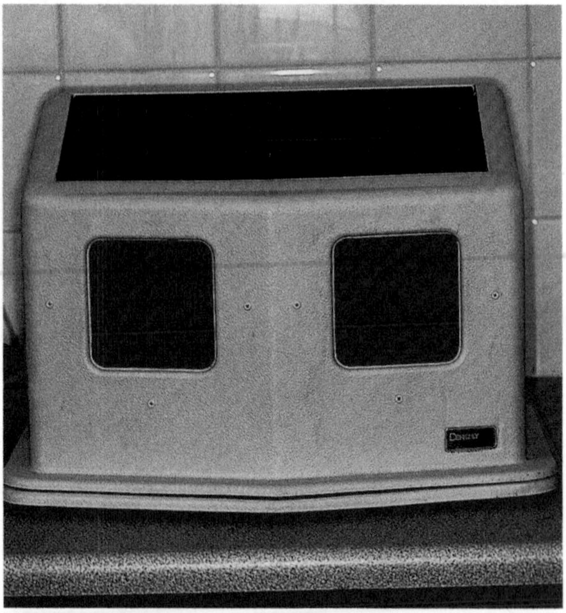

Fig. 7.5 The Rinn box. A chair-side 'darkroom' (Rinn box, manufactured by Dentsply) for processing dental film is a simple and inexpensive way of processing dental film. After processing in the Rinn box, thorough rinsing under running water (rubbing the film gently with your fingers, until it no longer feels 'soapy') is essential to avoid fixation stains.

Handling, mounting and viewing of dental radiographs

It is important to handle and mount processed dental films with care. Fingerprints can damage the emulsion on the film surface and the film is easily scratched. After rinsing thoroughly, adequate time should be allowed for the film to dry before being mounted or else it will adhere to the mount. It is also important to archive the film in such a way that it can be easily retrieved and identifiable. Remember that these films make up part of the patient's clinical records.

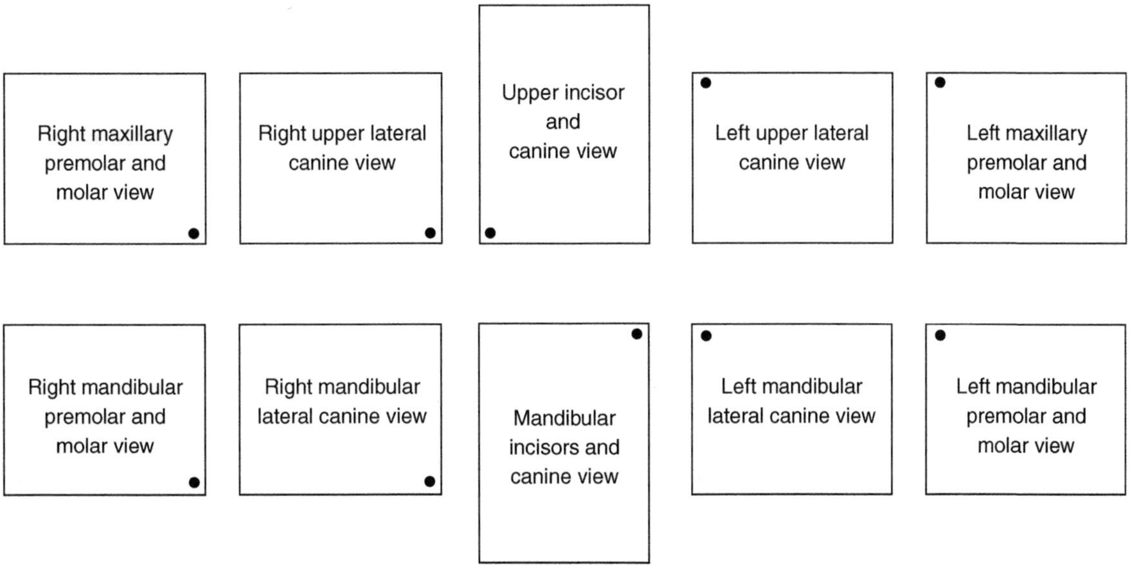

Fig. 7.6 Mounting if films exposed with dot facing forward in the mouth. Dental radiographs are viewed and mounted as if you were facing the animal and looking into its mouth. The raised dot should face you when viewing the film. Based on the anatomy of the jaws and teeth, it is then possible to identify upper and lower jaw views. If the films are always exposed with the dot facing forward in the mouth, then all views on the right side will have the dot in a different position from the left side views. This diagram depicts how we would mount a full mouth series of cat radiographs when all the films have been exposed with the dot facing forward. This is our preferred method.

Dental radiographs are viewed and mounted as if you were facing the animal and looking into its mouth. The raised dot should face you when viewing the film. Based on the anatomy of the jaws and teeth, it is then possible to identify upper and lower jaw views. If the films were always exposed with the dot facing forward in the mouth, then the views on the right side will have the dot in a different position from the left side views (Fig. 7.6). If the films were always exposed with the dot in the same position, then all the views on one side will have the dot on the distal aspect of the teeth and the views on the other side will have it on the mesial aspect of the teeth (Fig. 7.7).

PREPARATION OF THE PATIENT

General anaesthesia is required for dental radiography. Ideally, clinical examination and recording should precede the radiographic evaluation. It is also useful to clean the teeth before any radiographs are taken. Dental calculus, because it is radiodense, can obscure pathological lesions on a radiograph. The sequence is thus:

1. Examination and recording
2. Supragingival scaling
3. Radiography

INTRAORAL RADIOGRAPHIC TECHNIQUES

The film is placed intraorally and the incident beam directed through the tooth onto the film. The simplest way to hold the film in position is to place packing (foam wedge, swabs) behind it to sandwich the film against the tooth (Fig. 7.8). Various film holders are available but they can be difficult to use effectively.

The film should not be bent as this will lead to distortion of the image, resulting in either shortening or elongation of all or part of the tooth. If it does bend, a tongue spatula inserted below it is usually sufficient to stabilise the film. It should be borne in mind that superimposition of dental

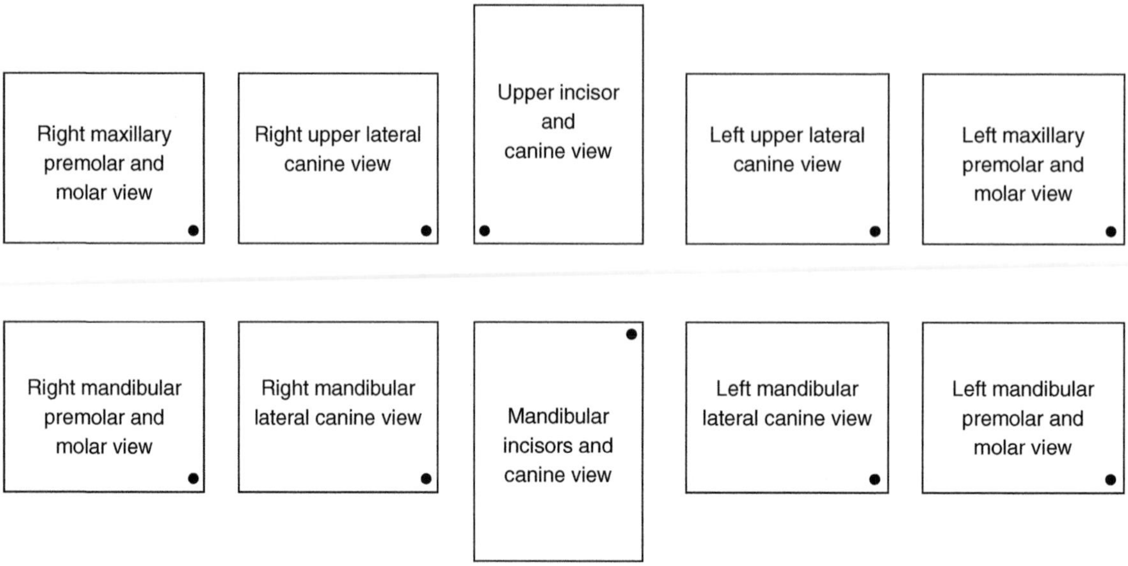

Fig. 7.7 Mounting if films exposed with the dot in the same position. If the films are always exposed with the dot in the same position, then all the views on one side will have the dot on the distal aspect of the teeth and the views on the other side will have it on the mesial aspect of the teeth. This diagram depicts how we would mount a full mouth series of cat radiographs if the films had been exposed with the dot always in the same position.

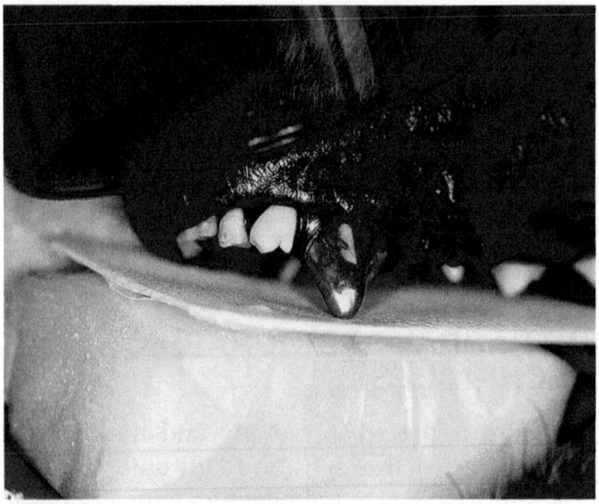

Fig. 7.8 Intraoral film placement. The simplest way to hold a film in position in the oral cavity is to insert packing (in this case a pack of swabs) behind it to sandwich the film against the tooth. The pack should be replaced for each animal.

structures will also lead to the creation of artefacts and hence the meticulous positioning for each tooth is worth the time taken. The three-rooted teeth (4th premolars and molars in the upper jaw) have an added consideration, namely the palatal root. In these teeth it is necessary to position the incident beam in such a way as to prevent superimposition of one root over another. Magnification is inevitable but keeping the film as close to the tooth as possible will minimise this. Changing the film–focus distance will also affect magnification.

The parallel technique is used to radiograph the mandibular premolars and molars. In this technique, the film is placed parallel to the teeth and the incident beam strikes the film perpendicularly. All other teeth are radiographed using the bisecting angle technique. In this technique, the acute angle created by the tooth axis and the film is bisected and the incident beam is directed perpendicular to this line.

The parallel technique

The parallel technique is used for the mandibular premolars and the molars. The patient is placed in lateral recumbency (with the side to be radiographed uppermost). The film is placed between the tongue and the teeth and pushed as far down into the sublingual fossa as possible. The X-ray beam is then directed from lateral to

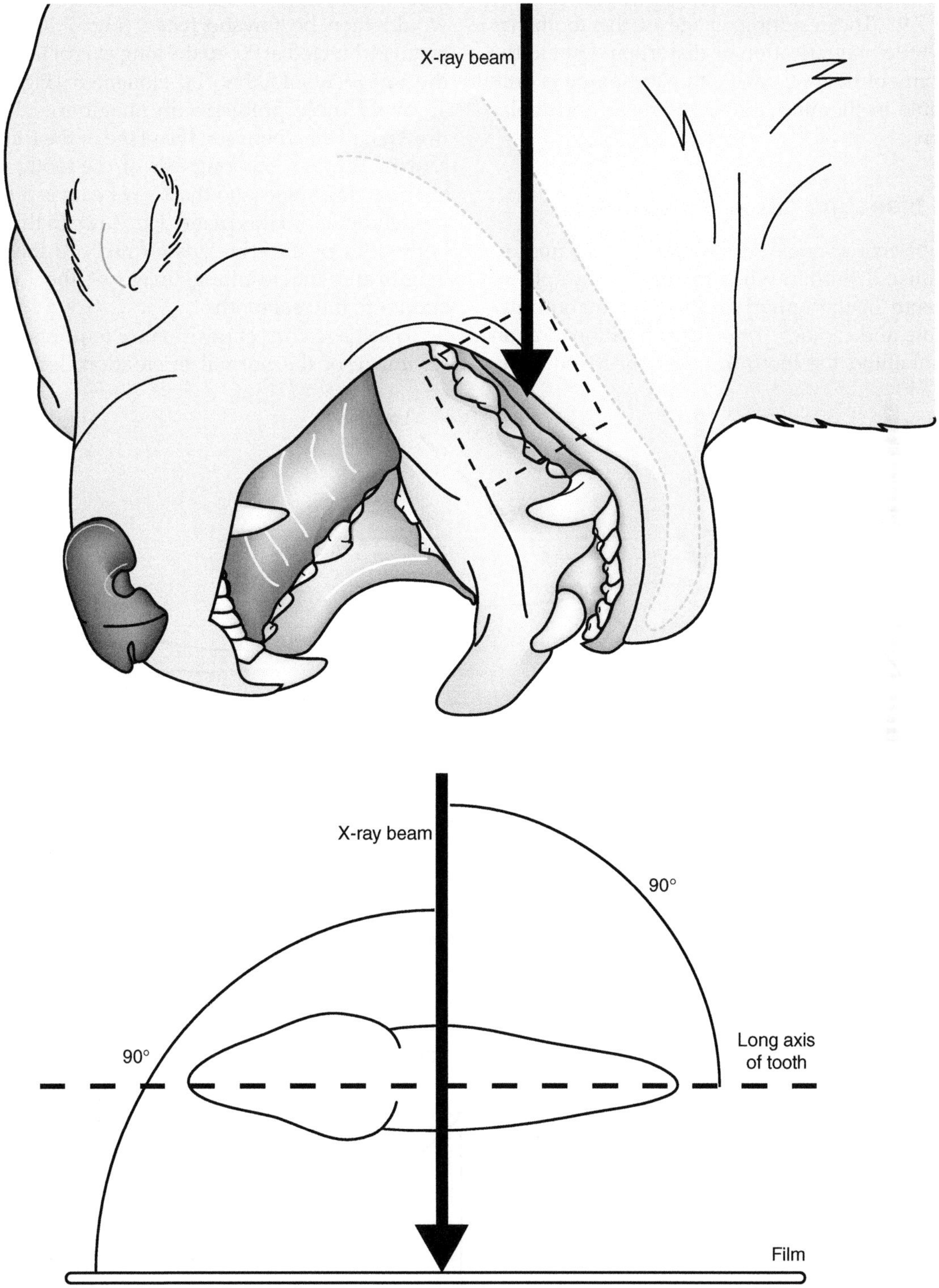

Fig. 7.9 The parallel technique. With the patient in lateral recumbency (with the side to be radiographed uppermost), the film is placed between the tongue and the teeth and pushed as far down into the sublingual fossa as possible. The X-ray beam is then directed from lateral to medial at right angles to the long axis of the tooth, which is parallel with the film.

medial at right angles to the long axis of the tooth (Fig. 7.9). The resulting image of the tooth has very little magnification or distortion. Due to the anatomy of the oral cavity, this technique is only possible in the mandibular premolar and molar regions.

The bisecting angle technique

The bisecting angle technique is required to minimise distortion when taking radiographs of the teeth in the upper jaw and the mandibular incisors and canines. The film is positioned at an angle behind the tooth in question. If the X-ray beam is directed at 90° to the film; the image would then be foreshortened (Fig. 7.10). If the beam is directed at 90° to the long axis of the tooth, the image would then be elongated (Fig. 7.11). To avoid these problems an imaginary plane is drawn half way between the plane of the film and a plane through the long axis of the tooth, i.e. at the bisecting angle, and the X-ray beam is directed perpendicular to this plane (Fig. 7.12). In this way, both sides of the triangles formed are the same length and the resulting image of the tooth is similar to the real tooth.

To achieve correct positioning requires a mental image of the normal orientation, length and

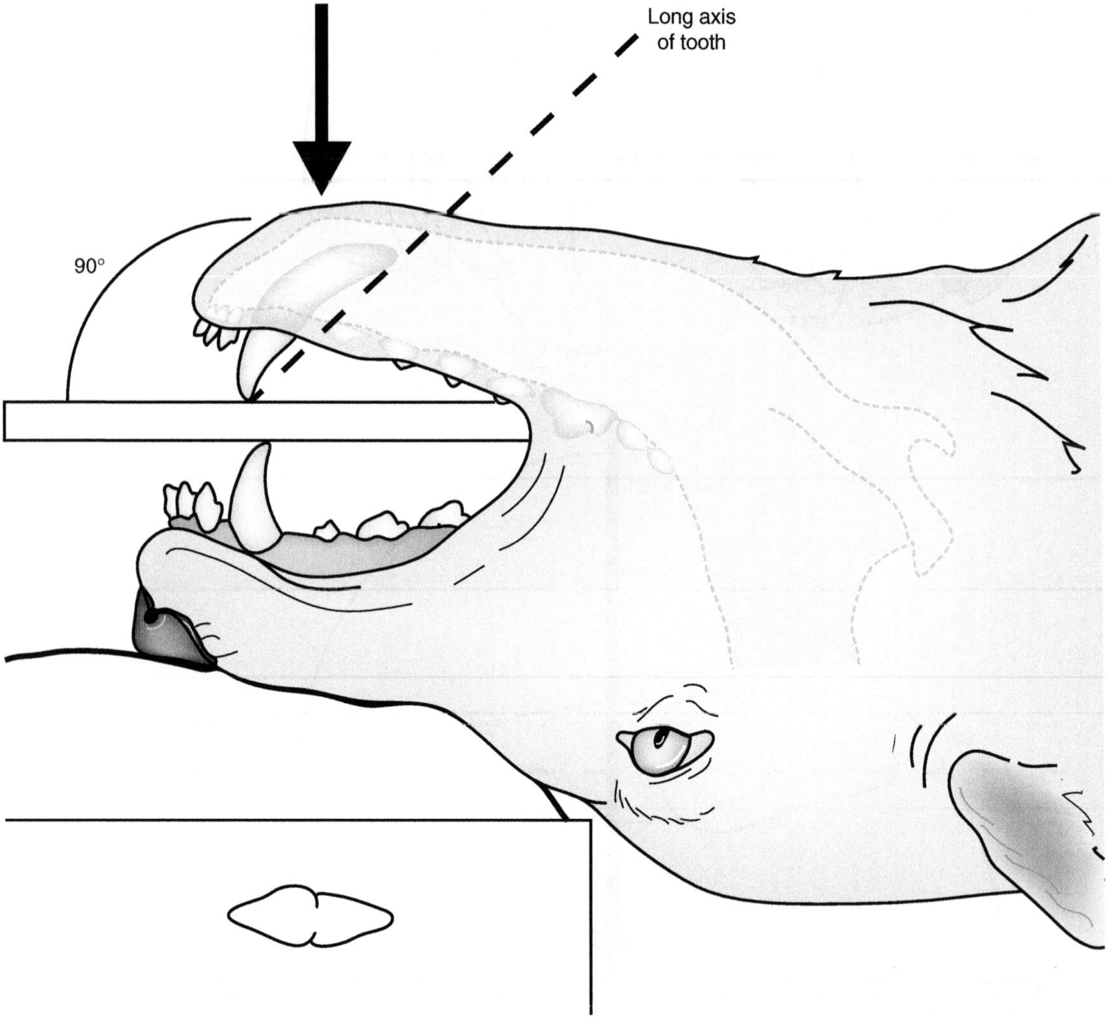

Fig. 7.10 Foreshortening of the image. If the X-ray beam is directed at 90° to the film, the image is foreshortened.

morphology of the tooth roots. Two tongue spatulas, fingers or instrument handles can be used to visualise these planes outside the mouth and so aid the positioning of the beam. A common problem is to 'miss the apex' of a tooth (especially on canine teeth) due to poor estimation of root length or position.

It may be helpful to position the patient as follows:

- Sternal recumbency for the incisors in the upper jaw
- Lateral or sternal recumbency for the canines, premolars and molars in the upper jaw
- Dorsal recumbency for the mandibular incisors
- Dorsal or lateral recumbency for mandibular canines

The premolar and molar views of the upper jaw of the cat are difficult. Often the zygomatic arch is superimposed over the roots and apices of the teeth. Placing a foam wedge or small sandbag under the nose, thus tilting the head up so that the dental arch is parallel with the table, will help avoid this.

Another common problem (in both dogs and cats) is superimposition of the mesiobuccal and mesiopalatal roots of the upper 4th premolar. It

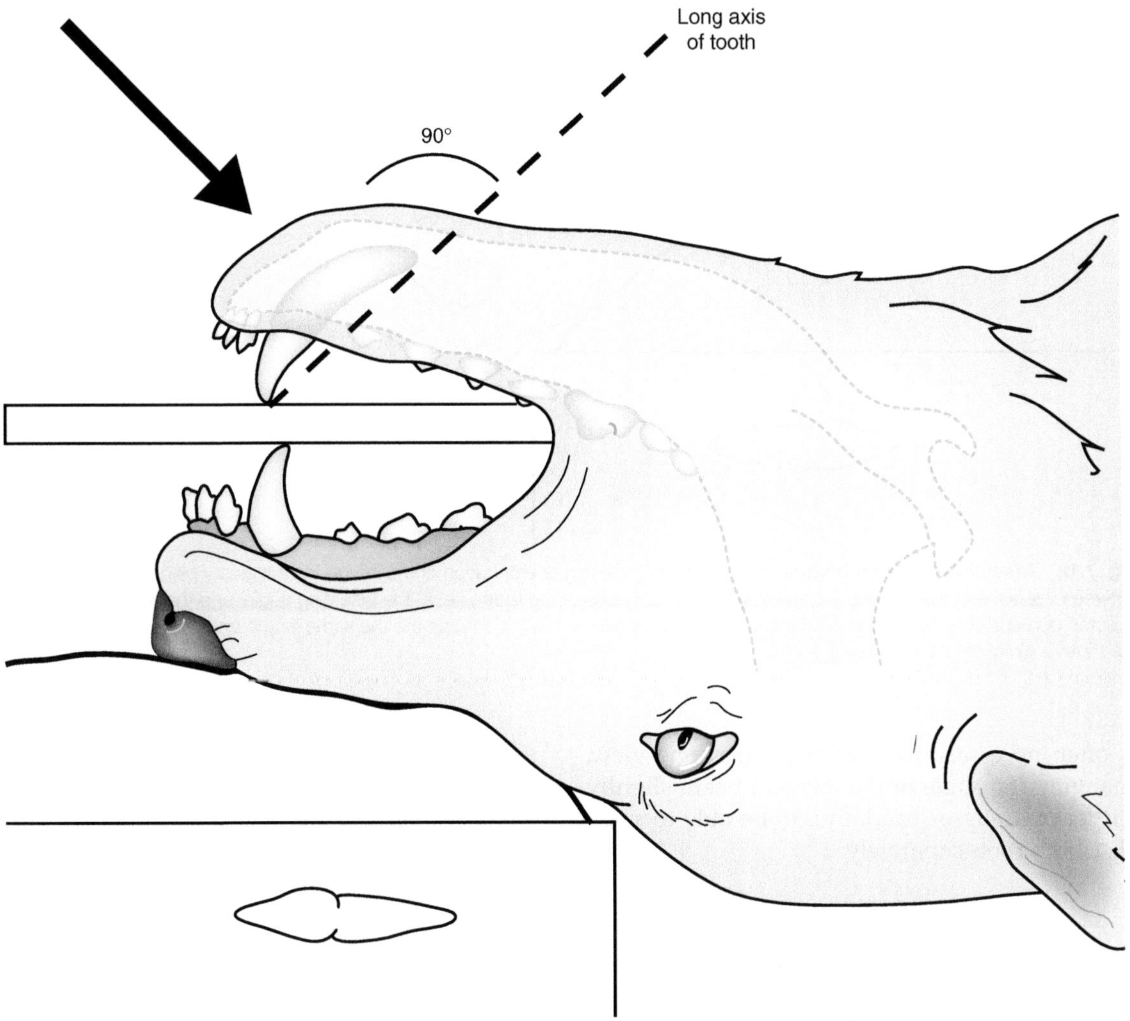

Fig. 7.11 Elongation of the image. If the beam is directed at 90° to the long axis of the tooth, the image is elongated.

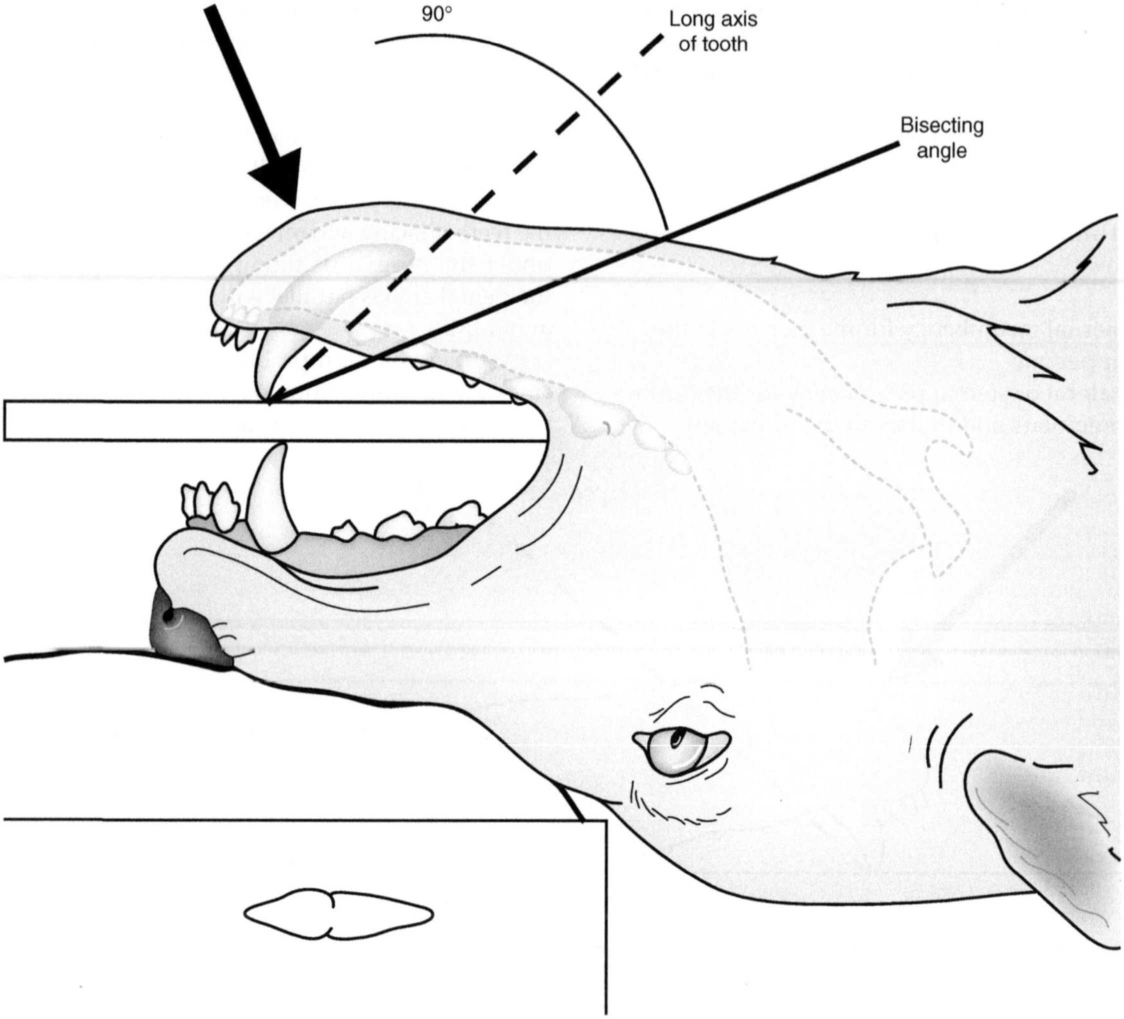

Fig. 7.12 Bisecting angle technique. To avoid foreshortening or elongation of the image, an imaginary plane is drawn half way between the plane of the film and a plane through the long axis of the tooth, i.e. at the bisecting angle, and the X-ray beam is directed perpendicular to this plane. In this way, both sides of the triangle formed are the same length and the resulting image of the tooth is similar to the real tooth.

is often necessary to take more than one view, changing the angle of the incident beam slightly (either rostrally or caudally), to be able to visualise both roots separately.

EXTRAORAL FILM PLACEMENT

When intraoral dental radiography is not available, extraoral views of the teeth may have to be used. Extraoral views are not ideal for dental examination mainly due to superimposition of the contralateral side, which obscures the image and causes distortion of the image. However, it may be possible to obtain diagnostic radiographs of the maxillary and mandibular premolars and molars using extraoral film placement, especially in dogs with wide skulls. Some examiners routinely use extraoral film placement to radiograph the maxillary premolars and molars in the cat.

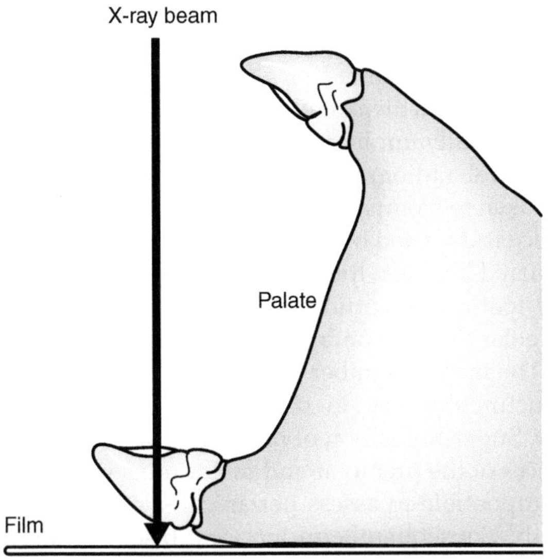

Fig. 7.13 Extraoral film placement. The film is placed on the table and the animal is placed in dorsolateral recumbency with the side to be radiographed closest to the film, i.e. the lower side of the animal's head. The mouth is held wide open using a radiolucent device, e.g. plastic needle cap. Tilting the head rotates the contralateral side away and an open mouth should mean the beam passes only through the soft tissue of the contralateral side. The tilting will place maxillary teeth almost parallel to the film, but the beam still requires adjustment according to the bisecting angle technique to reduce image distortion.

The technique is depicted in Figure 7.13. The film is placed on the table and the animal is placed in dorsolateral recumbency with the side to be radiographed closest to the film, i.e. the lower side of the animal's head. The mouth is held wide open using a radiolucent device, e.g. plastic needle cap. Tilting the head rotates the contralateral side away and an open mouth should mean the beam passes only through the soft tissue of the contralateral side. The tilting will place maxillary teeth almost parallel to the film but in reality the beam still requires adjustment according to the bisecting angle technique to reduce image distortion.

THE PARALLAX EFFECT

As a radiograph is two-dimensional, it is not possible to tell which of two objects in the image is nearer to the viewer. It is often necessary to know at what depth an object is, for example in locating an ectopic unerupted tooth. When a second image is taken, after rotating the beam position around the object's axis, the image of the object will move relative to other structures. When the object appears to move in the same direction as the shift in the X-ray head, it is placed lingually (nearer to the film); if it moves in the opposite direction it is more buccally positioned (further from the film). This technique is also useful to separate and identify two overlying roots, e.g. the mesiobuccal and palatal roots of an upper carnassial tooth in carnivores.

The SLOB rule (same direction lingual, opposite direction buccal) may help you remember the parallax effect. To use the SLOB rule you need to know the original and second beam position. An object that has moved in the same direction as you have moved the incident beam is lingually located. Conversely, an object that has moved in the opposite direction of that in which the incident beam has been moved is buccally located.

FULL MOUTH RADIOGRAPHS

Full mouth radiographs describes a series of films where each tooth of the dentition is accurately depicted in at least one view. A full mouth radiographic series of all animals undergoing dental examination provides valuable information, but is not always practically or financially viable. However, it is strongly recommended that all adult cats have full mouth radiographs taken as part of the oral and dental examination. Odontoclastic resorptive lesions are common in cats and clinical examination without radiography will only detect end-stage lesions.

In cats, it is necessary to take a minimum of 8 views, but 10 views are recommended, to ensure that all teeth are properly visualised. These are as follows:

Essential

- Incisor and canine view in the upper jaw
- Lateral view for each of the canines of the upper jaw
- Left and right maxillary premolar and molar views

- Mandibular incisor and canine view
- Left and right mandibular premolar and molar views

Recommended

- Lateral view for each of the canines of the mandible (in addition to the 8 essential views)

The choice of film size for each view is subjective. The smallest film that will depict the area of interest should be used to facilitate film positioning. We use adult periapical size film for all cat views.

In the case of dogs, full mouth radiographs are encouraged, especially at first examination. If this is not possible (time or financial restrictions) then radiographs are taken where indicated based on the findings during the clinical examination. In the event of full mouth radiographs, the size of film and the number of films used will depend upon the breed of dog and the shape of its face.

NORMAL RADIOGRAPHIC ANATOMY

The teeth and their supporting tissues

The component structures of the tooth and its supporting tissues are usually well defined radiographically (Fig. 7.2). The enamel of the tooth is seen as a very radiodense band that covers the crown and tapers to a fine edge at the cervical margin of the tooth. The enamel of the dog and cat is very much thinner than in humans and is often incompletely visualised on radiographs. The dentine is less radiodense than enamel and accounts for the bulk of the hard tissues of the mature tooth. The cementum, which covers the surface of the root of the tooth, is even less radiodense than dentine and is usually only visible when it has undergone hyperplasia. The pulp cavity, i.e. pulp chamber and the root canal(s), are visualised as a continuous radiolucent space in the centre of the tooth that extends from the coronal portion to the apex of the root(s). The size and width of the pulp chamber and root canal(s) will vary with the age of the animal. The lamina dura represents the bony wall of the tooth socket. It is seen as a radiodense line, which runs parallel to the root of the tooth. The lamina dura is not always visible on radiographs but a break in the path of a visible lamina dura usually implies periodontal pathology. Contralateral radiographs, however, should always be taken for comparison. The periodontal ligament space is depicted by a fine radiolucent line that is situated between the lamina dura and the root of the tooth. The cortical bone on the crest of the alveolar ridge is continuous with the lamina dura.

The largest number and variety of anatomical structures appear in radiographs of the upper jaw. Superimposition of nasal structures over the apices of the premolar and molar roots will make it impossible to assess periapical status of these teeth. Consequently an intraoral bisecting angle technique to avoid superimposition and give an accurate reproduction of the teeth is required in most instances.

Nutrient canals

The nutrient canals referred to here are those that contain blood vessels and nerves that supply the teeth, interdental spaces and gingiva. In radiographs, these are seen as radiolucent lines of uniform width, which sometimes have radiodense borders. The most easily identified nutrient canal is the mandibular canal, particularly the portion of it that extends from the mandibular foramen to the mental foramina (Fig. 7.2). Nutrient canals that arise from the mandibular canal are those that extend upward into the interdental space, and those that extend directly to the periapical foramina at the root of the tooth. Other nutrient canals that may be seen are the canal or groove that occupies the posterior superior alveolar artery and the anterior palatine (incisive) canal.

Foramina

Foramina may sometimes be mistaken for periapical lesions. Important foramina to remember are: the anterior palatine (incisive) foramen, the infraorbital foramina and the mental foramina.

Summary

- Radiography is mandatory for good dental practice
- Intraoral technique, employing parallel and bisecting angle views, is essential for meaningful results to be obtained
- Dental X-ray machines, with 'chair-side' processors, are ideal and such equipment proves convenient and cost-effective in most situations
- Full mouth radiographs are strongly advocated in cats in order to detect odontoclastic resorptive lesions. The technique is recommended in dogs also

FURTHER READING

Gorrel, C. (1998) Radiographic evaluation. In: Holmstrom, S. (ed) *Canine Dentistry. Veterinary Clinics of North America: Small Animal Practice*. Philadelphia: WB Saunders, pp. 1089–1110.

Gracis, M. & Harvey, C.E. (1998) Radiographic study of the maxillary canine tooth in metacephalic dogs. *Journal of Veterinary Dentistry* **15**(2): 73–78.

Robinson, J. & Gorrel, C. (1995) Oral examination and radiography. In: Crossley, D.A. & Penman, S. (eds) *Manual of Small Animal Dentistry*. Cheltenham: BSAVA, Ch. 5, pp. 35–49.

8

Periodontal disease

Periodontal disease is a collective term for a number of plaque-induced inflammatory lesions that affect the periodontium. It is the most common oral disease seen in dogs (Hamp et al, 1984). It is also common in the cat (Reichart et al, 1984). In fact, periodontal disease is probably the most common disease seen in small animal practice, with the great majority of dogs and cats over the age of three years having a degree of disease that warrants intervention.

Gingivitis is inflammation of the gingiva and is the earliest sign of disease. Individuals with untreated gingivitis *may* develop periodontitis. The inflammatory reactions in periodontitis result in destruction of the periodontal ligament and alveolar bone. The result of untreated periodontitis is ultimately exfoliation of the affected tooth. Thus, gingivitis is inflammation that is not associated with destruction (loss) of supporting tissue. It is reversible. In contrast, periodontitis is inflammation where the tooth has lost a variable degree of its support (attachment). It is generally irreversible. The salient features of gingivitis and periodontitis are depicted in diagrammatic form in Figure 8.1.

Periodontal disease can cause discomfort to affected individuals. Moreover, there is strong circumstantial evidence that a focus of infection in the oral cavity may cause disease of distant organs (DeBowes et al, 1996). Consequently, prevention and treatment of periodontal disease is important for the general health of companion animals. It is not a cosmetic issue! Prevention of periodontal disease is detailed in Chapter 10. This chapter details aetiology, pathogenesis, identification and treatment of periodontal disease.

AETIOLOGY

The *primary cause* of gingivitis and periodontitis is accumulation of *dental plaque* on the tooth surfaces. Periodontal disease is a unique infection in that it is not associated with a massive bacterial invasion of the tissues. Instead, the bacteria are localised to the hard surfaces of the tooth. Contrary to common belief, calculus (tartar) is only a secondary aetiological factor.

Dental plaque

Dental plaque is a biofilm composed of aggregates of bacteria and their by-products, salivary components, oral debris and occasional epithelial and inflammatory cells (Fig. 8.2). Plaque accumulation starts within minutes on a clean tooth surface. The formation of plaque involves two processes, namely the initial adherence of bacteria and then the continued accumulation of bacteria due to a combination of multiplication of bacteria and further aggregation of bacteria to those cells that are already attached. As soon as a tooth becomes exposed to the oral cavity, its surfaces are covered by the pellicle (an amorphous coating of salivary

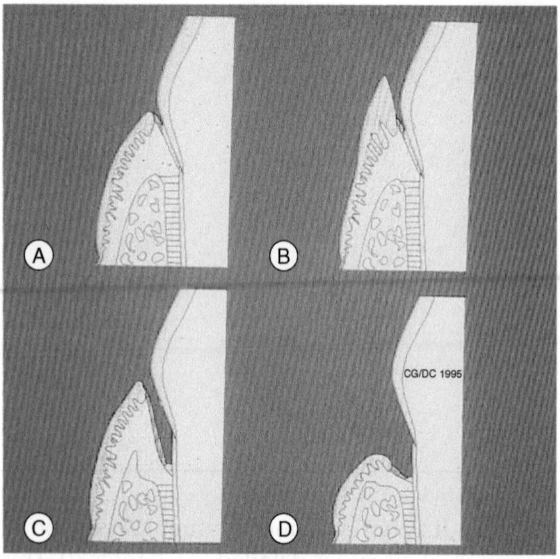

Fig. 8.1 Periodontal disease. Periodontal disease is a collective term for plaque-induced inflammation of the periodontium.

A: *Gingivitis*. The inflammation is limited to the gingiva, with no associated destruction of the periodontium. Gingivitis is reversible.

B: *Gingival hyperplasia*. Gingival hyperplasia may be the result of plaque-induced inflammation (hyperplastic gingivitis), but may also be of idiopathic or familial origin. It can also be induced by certain drugs. Gingival hyperplasia results in increased periodontal probing depths, initially with no loss of periodontal support, i.e. there is no attachment loss.

C: *Periodontitis with vertical bone destruction*. The plaque-induced inflammation results in irreversible destruction of the periodontal ligament and alveolar bone. The junctional epithelium (epithelial attachment) migrates apically and attaches on the root surfaces. If the gingival margin does not recede, the apical migration of the epithelial attachment results in increased periodontal probing depth, i.e. a pathological pocket is formed. Destruction of the alveolar bone can be horizontal or vertical. Shown here is vertical bone loss, resulting in the formation of a periodontal pocket where the apical extension of the pocket is below the margin of the alveolar bone, i.e. an infra-bony pocket.

D: *Periodontitis (with horizontal bone destruction)*. The periodontal destruction is evidenced by loss of periodontal ligament and horizontal bone loss. The junctional epithelium has migrated apically and attached to the root surfaces. However, the gingival margin has receded, so periodontal probing depths do not increase.

(Reproduced from the *Manual of Small Animal Dentistry* with kind permission of BSAVA.)

proteins and glycoproteins). The pellicle alters the charge and free energy of the tooth surfaces, which increases the efficiency of bacterial adhesion. Specific bacteria such as *Streptococcus sanguis* and *Actinomyces viscosus* can adhere to the pellicle. These bacteria produce extracellular polysaccharides, which aggregate other bacteria that are not otherwise able to adhere.

The initial accumulation of plaque occurs supragingivally but will extend into the sulcus and populate the subgingival region if left undisturbed. As demonstrated in a study where dogs were fed by intubation, the formation of dental plaque occurs whether food passes through the oral cavity or not, i.e. food debris does not attach to the teeth to form plaque (Egelberg, 1965). Supragingival plaque bacteria derive their main nutrients from dietary particles dissolved in saliva. Within the sulcus or pathological periodontal pocket, the major nutritional source for bacterial metabolism comes from the periodontal tissues and blood.

Classic experiments have demonstrated that accumulation of plaque on the tooth surfaces reproducibly induces an inflammatory response in associated gingival tissues, and that removal of the plaque leads to disappearance of the clinical signs of this inflammation (Löe et al, 1965; Theilade et al, 1966). Two hypotheses have been proposed to explain how plaque incites the inflammatory reactions in the periodontium. In the *non-specific plaque hypothesis* (Theilade, 1986), a direct relationship is assumed to exist between the total number of bacteria that accumulate on a tooth surface and the amplitude of the pathogenic effect. In the *specific plaque hypothesis* (Loesche, 1979), the view is that periodontitis is caused by specific pathogens (periodontopathogens). This hypothesis is supported by the fact that not all gingivitis lesions invariably develop to periodontitis lesions. However, differences in the composition of the subgingival plaque can be attributed in part to the local availability of blood products, pocket depth, redox potential and Po_2. Therefore, the question of whether the presence of specific microorganisms in patients or distinct sites may be the cause or consequence of disease is still a matter of dispute (Socransky et al, 1987). Many proposed periodontopathogens are strict anaerobes and, as such, may contribute little to the initiation of periodontitis in shallow periodontal pockets. Instead, these organisms are linked to

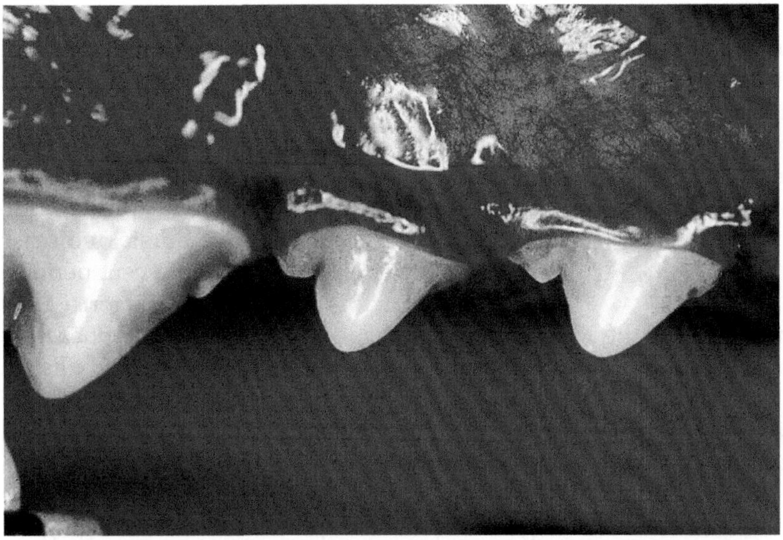

Fig. 8.2 Dental plaque. Dental plaque is a biofilm composed of aggregates of bacteria and their by-products, salivary components, oral debris and occasional epithelial and inflammatory cells. It starts accumulating within minutes on a clean tooth surface. Plaque may be difficult to see with the naked eye and the use of plaque-disclosing solutions (dye that stains plaque) is recommended for visualisation.

progression of disease in sites with pre-existing periodontitis.

As already mentioned, there is always plaque on the tooth surfaces. Plaque starts accumulating as soon as a tooth erupts into the oral cavity and within minutes of cleaning. The plaque associated with healthy gingiva is mainly comprised of aerobic and facultative anaerobic bacteria. As gingivitis develops, plaque extends subgingivally. Aerobes consume oxygen and a low redox potential is created, which makes the environment more suitable for growth of anaerobic species. The aerobic population does not decrease, but with an increasing number of anaerobes, the aerobic: anaerobic ratio decreases. The subgingival flora associated with periodontitis is predominantly anaerobic and consists of *Porphyromonas* spp., *Prevotella* spp., *Peptostreptococcus* spp., *Fusobacterium* spp. and spirochaetes (Hennet & Harvey, 1991). High levels of *Porphyromonas* spp. and spirochaetes are consistently associated with progressive periodontitis in the dog. The bacterial flora of the normal feline gingival margin, as well as the bacteria found in subgingival plaque of cats with gingivitis and periodontitis, are similar to those found in humans and dogs under similar conditions (Love et al, 1990; Mallonee et al, 1988).

To summarise, the first bacteria to adhere to the pellicle are aerobic Gram-positive organisms. In dogs and cats, the main bacteria in supragingival plaque are *Actinomyces* and streptococci. As the plaque thickens, matures and extends further down the gingival sulcus, the environment becomes suitable for growth of anaerobic organisms, motile rods and spirochaetes.

Dental calculus

Dental calculus is mineralised plaque. However, a layer of plaque always covers calculus. Both supragingival and subgingival plaque becomes mineralised. Supragingival calculus per se does not exert an irritant effect on the gingival tissues. In fact, it has been shown in monkeys that a normal attachment may be seen between the junctional epithelium and calculus if the calculus surface had been disinfected using chlorhexidine (Listgarten & Ellegaard, 1973). It has also been shown that sterilised calculus may be encapsulated in connective tissue without causing marked inflammation or abscess formation (Allen & Kerr, 1965). It has been speculated that calculus may exert a detrimental effect on the soft tissue owing to its rough surface. However, it has clearly been established that surface roughness alone does not initiate gingivitis (Waerhaug, 1956). The main importance of calculus in periodontal disease thus seems to be its role as a plaque-retentive surface.

This is supported by well-controlled animal (Nyman et al, 1986) and clinical human (Mombelli et al, 1995; Nyman et al, 1988) studies that have shown that the removal of subgingival plaque on top of subgingival calculus will result in healing of periodontal lesions and the maintenance of healthy periodontal tissues.

PATHOGENESIS

The pathogenic mechanisms involved in the establishment of periodontal disease include:

- Direct injury by plaque bacteria
- Indirect injury by plaque bacteria via inflammation

As already mentioned, periodontal disease is rarely associated with invasion of the periodontal tissues by plaque bacteria. Moreover, many microbial products have little or no direct toxic effect on the host. However, they possess the potential to activate non-immune and immune inflammatory reactions that cause the tissue damage. It is now well accepted that *it is the host's response to the plaque bacteria, rather than microbial virulence per se, that causes the tissue damage* (Kinane & Lindhe, 1997).

In gingivitis, the plaque-induced inflammation is limited to the soft tissue of the gingiva (Fig. 8.1A). Sulcus depths are normal (i.e. periodontal probing depths are 1–3 mm in the dog and 0.5–1 mm in the cat). As periodontitis occurs (Fig. 8.1C), the inflammatory destruction of the coronal part of the periodontal ligament allows apical migration of the epithelial attachment and the formation of a pathological periodontal pocket (i.e. periodontal probing depths increase). If the inflammatory disease is permitted to progress, the crestal portion of the alveolar process begins to resorb. The type and extent of alveolar bone destruction is assessed radiographically. The resorption may proceed apically on a horizontal level. Horizontal bone destruction is often accompanied by gingival recession, so periodontal pockets may not form (Fig. 8.1D). If there is no gingival recession, the periodontal pocket is supra-alveolar, i.e. above the level of the alveolar margin. The pattern of bone destruction may also proceed in a vertical direction along the root to form angular bony defects. The periodontal pocket is now infra- or subalveolar, i.e. below the margin of the alveolar bone.

Disease progression is generally an episodic occurrence rather than a continuous process. Tissue destruction occurs as acute bursts of disease activity followed by relatively quiescent periods. The acute burst is clinically characterised by rapid deepening of the periodontal pocket as periodontal ligament fibres and alveolar bone are destroyed by the inflammatory reactions. The quiescent phase is not associated with clinical or radiographic evidence of disease progression. However, complete healing does not occur during this quiescent phase, because subgingival plaque remains on the root surfaces and inflammation persists in the connective tissue. The inactive phase can last for extended periods.

Other conditions, such as physical or psychological stress and malnutrition, may impair protective responses, such as the production of antioxidants and acute phase proteins, and can aggravate periodontitis but do not actually cause destructive tissue inflammation. A genetic predisposition to destructive inflammation of the periodontium may be important in some individuals. In humans, a strong association has been observed between the severity of periodontitis and a specific genotype of the interleukin-1 (IL-1) gene cluster (Kornman et al, 1997). Patients carrying this periodontitis-associated genotype (PAG) may demonstrate phenotypic differences, as indicated by elevated levels of IL-1β in gingival sulcular (crevicular) fluid (Engebretson et al, 1999). No similar data are available for the dog or cat.

Significance

Undisturbed plaque accumulation results in gingivitis. While some individuals with untreated gingivitis will develop periodontitis, not all animals with untreated gingivitis do so. It cannot be predicted which individuals with gingivitis will develop periodontitis. However, animals in which clinically healthy gingivae are maintained will not develop periodontitis. Consequently, *the aim in periodontal disease prevention and treatment is to establish and maintain clinically healthy gingivae to prevent periodontitis.*

ASSESSMENT OF PERIODONTAL STATUS

General considerations

Evidence of periodontal disease relies on clinical examination of the periodontium in the anaesthetised animal. In addition, radiography is mandatory if there is evidence of periodontitis on clinical examination. It is essential to differentiate between gingivitis and periodontitis in order to institute appropriate treatment. In individuals with gingivitis, the aim is to restore the tissues to clinical health; and in individuals with established periodontitis, the aim of therapy is to prevent progression of disease.

Oral examination and recording of findings are detailed in Chapter 6. The following parameters need to be assessed and recorded for *each tooth* in *all patients*:

1. Gingivitis and gingival index
2. Periodontal probing depth (PPD)
3. Gingival recession (GR)
4. Furcation involvement
5. Mobility

Periodontal probing depth, gingival recession, furcation involvement and mobility measure the extent of destruction of the periodontium, i.e. assess the presence and severity of periodontitis.

We do not assess and record the extent of plaque and calculus accumulation in patients that are seen for the first time. These deposits will be removed during periodontal therapy. Instead, we assess and record plaque at follow-up visits to assess the efficacy of the home care regimen that has been instituted. Plaque accumulation is visualised using a plaque-disclosing solution and the teeth that have plaque at the gingival margin are noted and recorded. The amount of plaque is graded subjectively as mild, moderate or severe depending on the depth of staining achieved by the plaque-disclosing solution.

Gingivitis

Gingivitis is defined as a *reversible* plaque-induced inflammation limited to the gingiva (i.e. no loss of periodontal attachment).

Clinical signs

Gingivitis manifests clinically as swelling, reddening and often bleeding of the gingival margin (Fig. 8.3). It may be accompanied by halitosis.

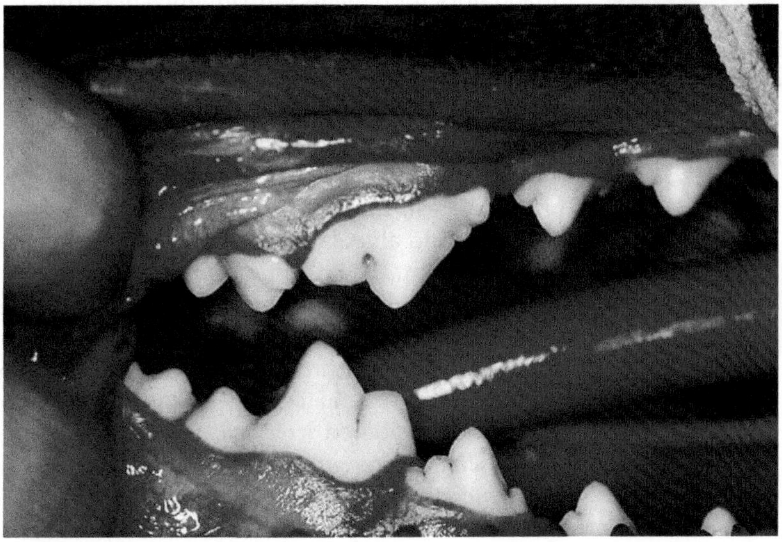

Fig. 8.3 Gingivitis. This manifests clinically as swelling and reddening of the gingival margin.

Assessment of gingivitis

The presence and degree of gingival inflammation is assessed based on a combination of redness and swelling, as well as presence or absence of bleeding on gentle probing of the gingival sulcus. Various indices can be used to give a numerical value to the degree of gingival inflammation present. In the clinical situation, a simple bleeding index is the most useful. Using this method, the gingival sulcus of each tooth is gently probed at several points and given a score of 0 if there is no bleeding and a score of 1 if the probing elicits bleeding. The patient with uncomplicated gingivitis will have normal periodontal probing depths (1–3 mm in the dog and 0.5–1 mm in the cat) and show no evidence of gingival recession, furcation involvement or tooth mobility. Radiography is not mandatory if the clinical examination reveals no evidence of periodontal destruction, i.e. periodontitis.

Gingival hyperplasia (Figs 8.1B and 8.4) may be the result of plaque-induced inflammation, i.e. hyperplastic gingivitis. It may also be of idiopathic or familial origin; and it can be induced by certain drugs, e.g. hydantoin, cyclosporins. Gingival hyperplasia is common in some breeds, e.g. boxer, springer spaniel. There is an increase in periodontal probing depths due to the gingival overgrowth.

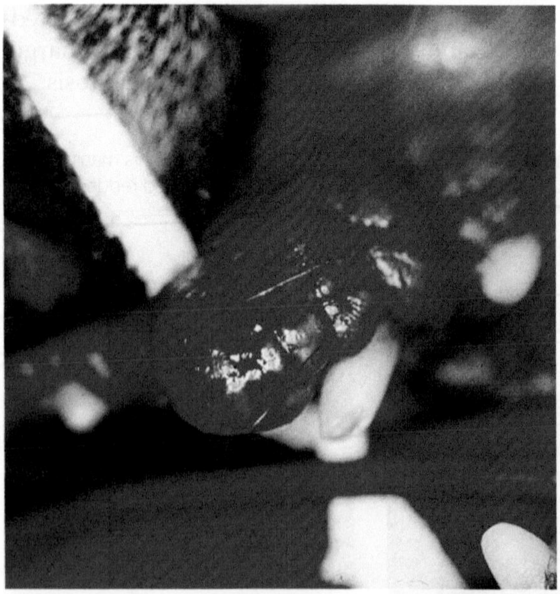

Fig. 8.4 Gingival hyperplasia. The hyperplastic gingival tissue almost covers the crowns, resulting in the formation of pseudopockets.

Consequences to affected animal

Uncomplicated gingivitis is generally not associated with discomfort or pain in humans. In fact, it is an insidious process and the patient may be unaware of its existence. The significance of gingivitis is that, if untreated, periodontitis may develop as described earlier.

Gingival hyperplasia does pose an additional concern. The hyperplastic gingiva alters the position of the gingival margin and results in a false or 'pseudo' pocket. It is called a pseudopocket, as the increased periodontal probing depth is not due to destruction of periodontal ligament and alveolar bone with apical migration of the junctional epithelium as in periodontitis. Instead, the increased periodontal probing depth is due to the overgrowth of the gingiva. However, the presence of hyperplastic gingiva compromises tooth cleaning and may predispose to periodontitis. If periodontitis develops, the increased periodontal probing depth is due to both gingival hyperplasia and loss of attachment. Consequently, radiography (to assess the status of the alveolar bone) is mandatory for patients with gingival hyperplasia.

Periodontitis

Individuals with untreated gingivitis *may* develop periodontitis. The inflammatory reactions in periodontitis result in destruction of the periodontal ligament and alveolar bone, i.e. loss of periodontal attachment. The result of untreated periodontitis is eventually exfoliation of the affected tooth. It is important to remember that periodontitis is a *site-specific disease*, i.e. it may affect one or more sites of one or several teeth. Periodontitis can generally be considered *irreversible. The aim of treatment is thus to prevent development of new lesions at other sites and to prevent further tissue destruction at sites that are already affected.*

Clinical signs

Halitosis is common and is often the first sign noted by the pet owner. Large amounts of dental deposits are usually present. These deposits need to be removed to allow a detailed examination of the periodontium. In severely affected cases, gingival recession, furcation involvement and tooth mobility may be evident on conscious examination. Ulcers affecting mucous membranes of lips and cheeks may be present in areas where these tissues are exposed to plaque-covered tooth surfaces (Fig. 8.5).

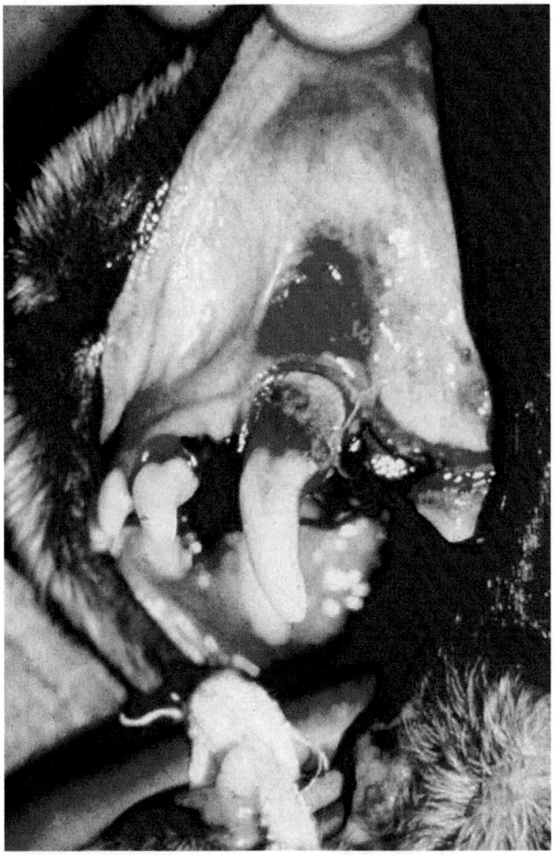

Fig. 8.5 Gingival recession and mucous membrane ulceration. The periodontal ligament and alveolar bone on the labial aspect of the left upper canine has been destroyed. The gingival margin has receded. Periodontal probing depth is 1 mm, i.e. there is no pathological pocket. A mucous membrane ulcer has developed on the lip surface that is in contact with the plaque-covered tooth surface. While uncomplicated periodontitis is not associated with severe discomfort, these mucous membrane ulcers are known to be painful!

Assessment of periodontitis

Tissue destruction in periodontitis is assessed by measuring periodontal probing depth, gingival recession, furcation involvement and degree of tooth mobility. In many cases, measuring or calculating the periodontal attachment level (PAL) is also useful. Periodontal probing depth is not necessarily correlated with severity of attachment loss (Fig. 8.6). Gingival hyperplasia may contribute to a deep pocket (or pseudopocket if there is no attachment loss), while gingival recession may result in the absence of a pocket but also minimal remaining attachment. Periodontal attachment level records the distance from the cemento-enamel junction (or from a fixed point on the tooth) to the base or apical extension of the pathological pocket. It is thus a more accurate assessment of tissue loss in periodontitis. PAL can either be measured with a periodontal probe or it can be calculated (e.g. PPD + gingival recession, or PPD − gingival hyperplasia).

Radiography to assess the type and extent of alveolar bone destruction is mandatory for periodontitis patients. Consequently, full mouth radiographs of periodontitis patients should be performed prior to the institution of any therapy. In addition, radiographs need to be taken at regular intervals to monitor outcome of any treatment. A detailed examination of the periodontal ligament space and interproximal alveolar margin requires the use of an intraoral radiographic technique (detailed in Ch. 7). The radiographic changes associated with periodontal disease include resorption of the alveolar margin, widening of the periodontal ligament space, a break in the path or loss of the radiopacity of the lamina dura and destruction of alveolar bone resulting in supra- or infra-bony pockets.

A periodontal abscess is an acute exacerbation of the process occurring in a chronic periodontal pocket (Fig. 8.7). It usually occurs from partial or complete obstruction of the orifice of the pocket. Multiple acute periodontal abscesses may occur in some cases of advanced generalised periodontitis. An abscess may also develop in the healthy periodontium if a foreign body is forced beyond the epithelial attachment. Grass seeds embedded

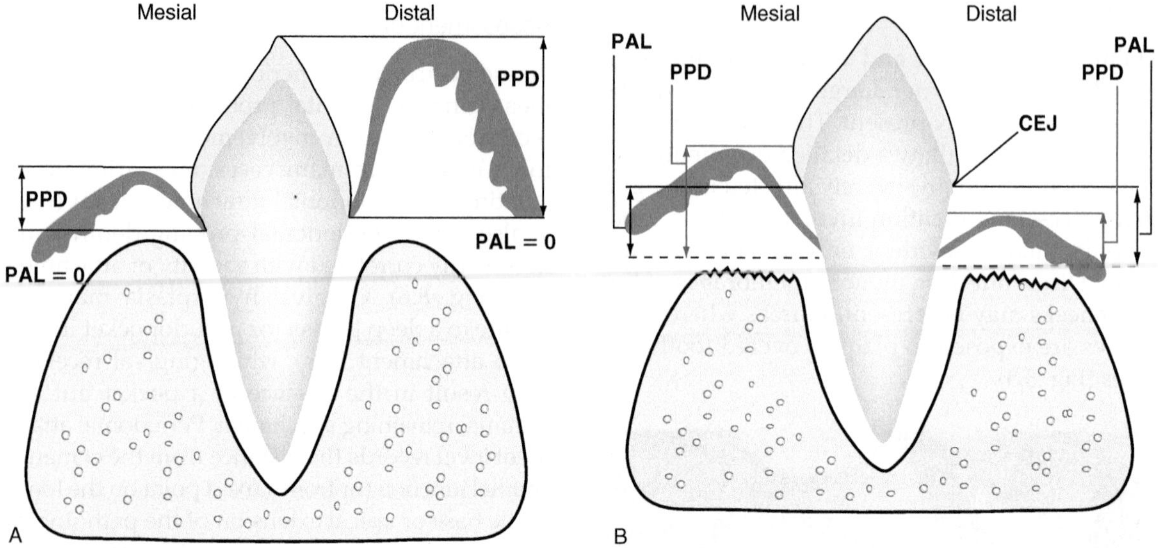

Fig. 8.6 Attachment loss.
A: The epithelial attachment on both sides of the tooth is at the cemento-enamel junction, so there is no loss of periodontal attachment (PAL = 0). The surface labelled mesial depicts normal gingival attachment, periodontal probing depth is 1–2 mm. The surface labelled distal has an increased periodontal probing depth, e.g. 8 mm due to gingival hyperplasia. However, this is not periodontitis as there has been no loss of periodontal support.
B: Periodontal probing depth on the surface labelled mesial is increased, e.g. 6 mm. Periodontal probing depth on the side labelled distal is normal, i.e. 1–2 mm, due to the gingival recession. Periodontal attachment loss, i.e. the extent of periodontal ligament and alveolar bone destruction is the same.

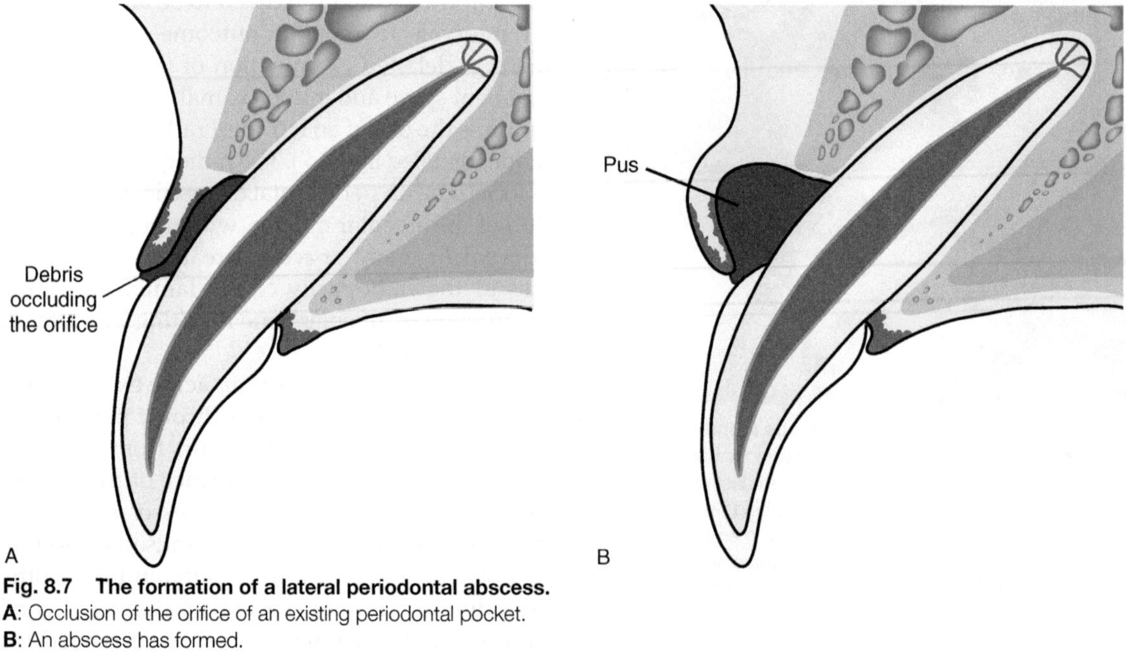

Fig. 8.7 The formation of a lateral periodontal abscess.
A: Occlusion of the orifice of an existing periodontal pocket.
B: An abscess has formed.

in the gingival sulcus have been identified as causing acute periodontal abscessation in the dog. The acute periodontal abscess may produce rapid and extensive bone loss. In some instances, the bone loss will extend beyond the apices of the roots of the teeth.

Consequences to affected animal

Based on feedback from human patients, uncomplicated periodontitis is not associated with severe pain or discomfort. In contrast, complications such as the development of a lateral periodontal abscess or ulcers in the mucous membranes are very painful.

It has been shown that a severe infection in the oral cavity, as with extensive periodontitis, will lead to a transient bacteraemia on chewing (Thoden van Velzen et al, 1984). In fact, an association has been demonstrated between periodontal disease and histopathological changes in kidney, myocardium and liver (DeBowes et al, 1996).

TREATMENT

General considerations

The treatment of periodontal disease is aimed at controlling the cause of the inflammation, i.e. dental plaque. Conservative or cause-related periodontal therapy consists of removal of plaque and calculus, and any other remedial procedures required, under general anaesthesia, in combination with daily maintenance of oral hygiene. In other words, the treatment of periodontal disease has two components:

- Maintenance of oral hygiene
- Professional periodontal therapy

Maintenance of oral hygiene is performed by the owner and is often called home care. Its effectiveness depends on the motivation and technical ability of the owner and the cooperation of the animal. Home care is detailed in Chapter 10. The veterinary nurse and technician have an important role to play in instituting and maintaining home care.

Professional periodontal therapy is performed under general anaesthesia and includes:

- Supra- and subgingival scaling
- Root planing
- Tooth crown polishing
- Subgingival lavage
- Periodontal surgery in selected cases

The term 'dental prophylaxis' or 'prophy' has been used to encompass clinical examination and professional periodontal therapy. This is misleading since the real prophylaxis, i.e. steps taken to prevent disease development and progression, is not the professional periodontal therapy carried out under general anaesthesia but the daily home care regime to remove plaque. If no home care is instituted, then plaque will rapidly reform after a professional periodontal therapy procedure and the disease will progress. Before any treatment is instituted, the owner must be made aware that home care is the most essential component in both preventing and treating periodontal disease. Whenever possible it is useful to institute a home care programme before any professional periodontal therapy is performed.

The aim of treatment differs depending on whether there is gingivitis only or periodontitis as well.

Gingivitis

Gingivitis is by definition reversible. Removal or adequate reduction of plaque will restore inflamed gingivae to health. Once clinically healthy gingivae have been achieved, these can be maintained by daily removal or reduction in the accumulation of plaque. In short, the treatment of gingivitis is to restore the inflamed tissues to clinical health and then to maintain clinically healthy gingivae (Fig. 8.8), thus preventing periodontitis. The purpose of the professional periodontal therapy in the gingivitis patient is removal of dental deposits, mainly calculus (which is not removed by toothbrushing). Once the teeth have been cleaned it remains up to the owner to remove the plaque that re-accumulates on a daily basis.

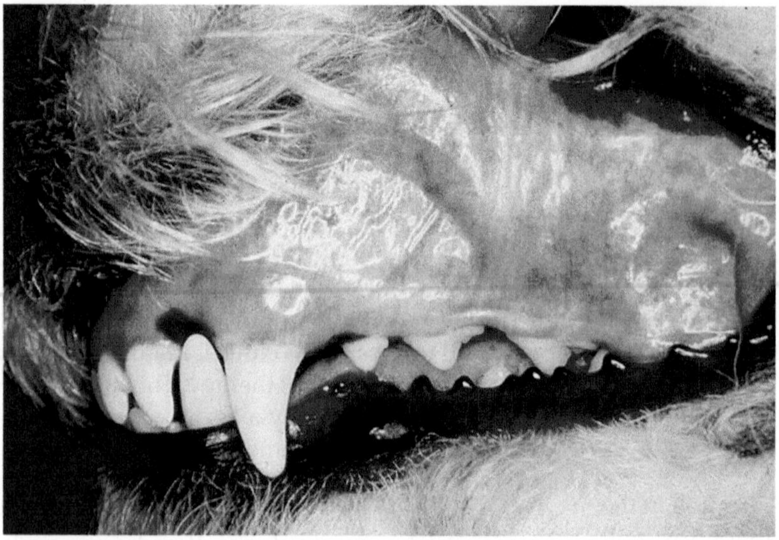

Fig. 8.8 Clinically healthy gingivae. With good home care, clinically healthy gingivae can be maintained for the lifespan of the animal. An animal with clinically healthy gingivae will not develop periodontitis.

Summary for treatment of gingivitis

- Educate the owner to understand the disease process
- Train and motivate the owner to perform daily home care
- Institute daily home care regimen by the owner – ideally, toothbrushing with a pet toothpaste in conjunction with a dental hygiene product
- Professional periodontal therapy (supra- and subgingival scaling and polishing) under general anaesthesia to remove dental deposits (plaque and calculus)
- Regular check-ups to ensure that the owner is following recommendations and to boost the owner's motivation

Periodontitis

Untreated gingivitis may progress to periodontitis. In most instances in a practice situation, periodontitis is irreversible. It is important to remember that periodontitis is a site-specific disease, i.e. it may affect one or more sites of one or several teeth. The aim of treatment is thus to prevent development of new lesions at other sites and to prevent further tissue destruction at sites that are already affected.

Professional periodontal therapy removes dental deposits above and below the gingival margin. It then rests with the owner to ensure that plaque does not re-accumulate. Meticulous supragingival plaque control, by means of daily toothbrushing and adjunctive antiseptics when indicated, will prevent migration of the plaque below the gingival margin. If the subgingival tooth surfaces are kept clean, the junctional epithelium will reattach.

In patients with suspected periodontitis (obvious furcation involvement, gingival recession, etc. on a conscious examination), it is useful to institute daily toothbrushing three to four weeks prior to the planned professional periodontal therapy if the animal will allow it. This will result in less inflamed tissue at the time of professional therapy and will allow assessment of the ability of the owner to perform home care. If home care is not possible, the professional treatment will need to be more radical.

Summary for treatment of periodontitis

- Educate the owner to understand the disease process
- Train and motivate the owner to perform daily home care
- Institute daily home-care regimen by the owner
- Professional periodontal therapy: this includes supra- and subgingival scaling and polishing, root planing and extraction of unsalvageable teeth under general anaesthesia
- Regular check-ups to ensure owner is following recommendations and to boost owner's motivation
- Periodontal surgery may be indicated

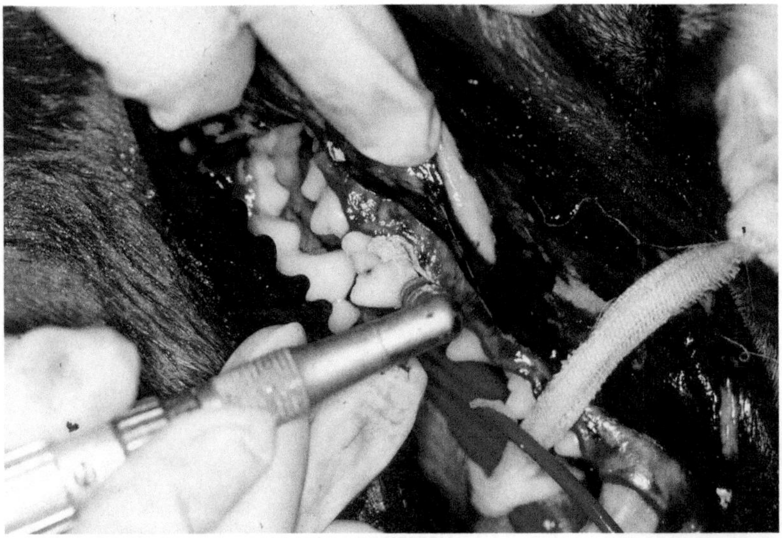

Fig. 8.9 How to hold dental instruments. Dental instruments are generally held using a modified pen grip as depicted here. Resting the 4th and 5th fingers on adjacent structures gives stability and support, reducing the risk of slippage and iatrogenic injuries.

PROFESSIONAL PERIODONTAL THERAPY

General considerations

Professional periodontal therapy must be performed under general anaesthesia. Anaesthetic monitoring and special care of the patient undergoing dentistry and/or oral surgery is covered in Chapter 3. The basic instrument requirements for periodontal therapy are covered in Chapter 2.

To master the technical skills required for dentistry and oral surgery, attending practical courses is recommended. In general, dental instruments are held in a modified pen grip (Fig. 8.9) and the 4th and 5th fingers are placed on adjacent structures (neighbouring teeth, opposite jaw) for stability and support.

The procedures

Supragingival scaling

Supragingival scaling is the removal of plaque and calculus above the gingival margin. It can be performed using hand instruments alone or a combination of hand instruments and powered scalers.

The recommended procedure is as follows:

- Remove gross dental deposits (plaque covered calculus) using rongeurs, extraction forceps or calculus-removing forceps (Fig. 8.10)

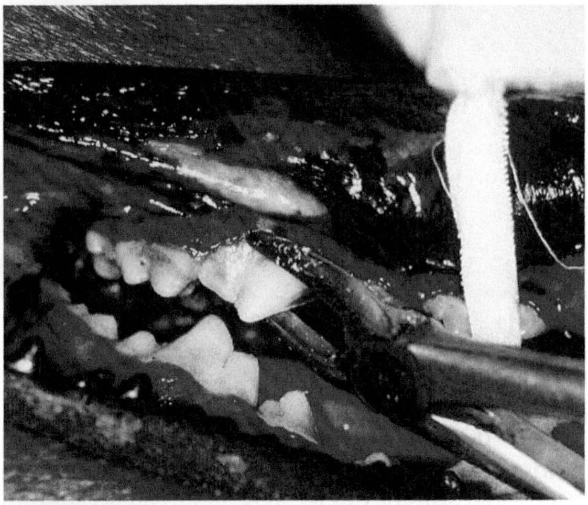

Fig. 8.10 Removing gross supragingival dental deposits with extraction forceps. Do not traumatise the gingival margin with the forceps.

- Remove residual supragingival dental deposits with sharp hand instruments (either a sickle-shaped scaler or a curette), as demonstrated in Figure 8.11
- A powered scaler (either an ultrasonic or a sonic scaler) is then used to remove residual dental deposits (Fig. 8.12)

Powered scalers generate heat and have the potential to cause iatrogenic damage if not used properly. Overheating a tooth will cause desiccation

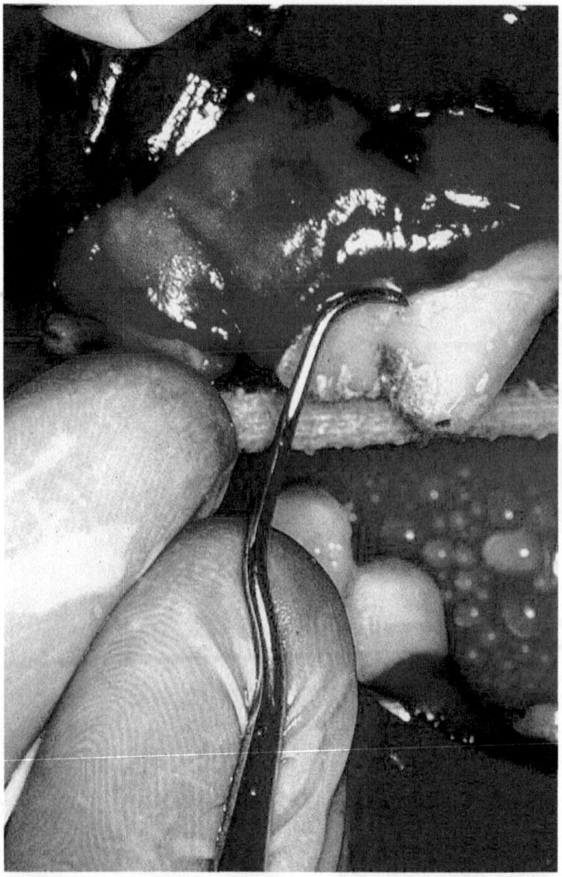

Fig. 8.11 Removing supragingival dental deposits with hand instruments. In this slide, a universal scaler is being used to remove calculus.

of the dentine and consequent damage to the underlying pulp tissue. Pulp damage may be a reversible pulpitis but it can become severe enough to cause pulp necrosis, which would necessitate extraction or endodontic treatment of the affected tooth.

An ultrasonic or sonic scaler should be used by gently stroking the tooth with the side of the tip and with continuous movement over the tooth surface. A plentiful supply of water is essential to cool the oscillating tip and flush away debris. Using the tip of the instrument or applying excessive pressure will cause gouging of the tooth surface as well as generating excessive heat. As an arbitrary rule, it is suggested that no more than 15 seconds of continuous scaling should be performed on any one tooth. If the tooth is not clean in that period of time, then return to it after scaling a few other teeth. This will allow the original tooth time to cool down.

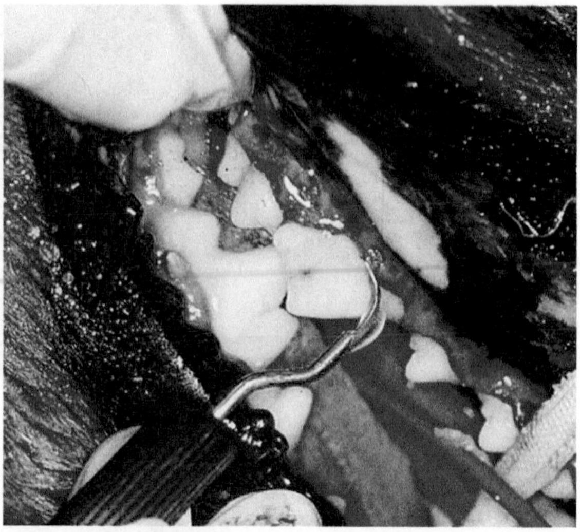

Fig. 8.12 Removing supragingival dental deposits with an ultrasonic scaler. The use of a fine perio (sickle, universal) insert is recommended for both ultrasonic and sonic scalers.

Both sonic and ultrasonic scalers should be used with a thin pointed tip, sometimes called a perio, sickle or universal insert. The large (wide) tip is not recommended. A fine tip will remove dental deposits more accurately, with less likelihood of damage to the tooth enamel.

Subgingival scaling and root planing

Subgingival scaling is the removal of plaque, calculus and other debris from the tooth surface below the gingival margin, i.e. within the gingival sulcus or periodontal pocket. There is no need to perform extensive subgingival scaling if there is no calculus below the gingival margin. However, the presence of subgingival deposits should always be investigated with a dental explorer and removed if any are identified. Root planing is the removal of the superficial layer of toxin-laden cementum from the root surfaces. Root planing produces a smooth root surface which is less likely to accumulate plaque and more likely to permit epithelial reattachment. Excessive root planing may damage the root surface (expose root dentine to the periodontal ligament) and predispose to further periodontal destruction. So, while a clean and smooth root surface should be obtained; overzealous root planing should be avoided.

The healing process after subgingival scaling and root planing is depicted diagrammatically in Figure 8.13B, C and D. Scaling and planing are achieved simultaneously using a curette. The procedure can be performed using either a closed (without raising an access flap) or open (raising an access flap) technique. An open technique is recommended for pockets deeper than 4 mm as it is difficult even for a skilled operator to ensure that all subgingival deposits have been removed without raising a gingival flap for direct access and visualisation. However, an open technique is only indicated in patients with proven sufficient home care, i.e. it is not first line treatment. The open technique is not a routine hygiene procedure. It is classified as periodontal surgery and should be performed by a veterinarian with expertise in veterinary dentistry.

Ultrasonic and sonic scalers are designed for supragingival work. Once inserted into the gingival sulcus or pathological pocket the water will no longer reach to cool the tip. This then results in thermal damage of both hard and soft tissues. Quick subgingival excursions are permissible only if the gingiva is oedematous, or held mechanically out of the way to allow the water to reach the tip. Scalers with specially designed working tips where the water exits at the very end are safer to use under the gingival margin, but the removal of established subgingival deposits can only be adequately performed with meticulous use of sharp curettes. The curette has a sharp working or cutting edge on the curved blade and has a rounded tip. Most curettes are double ended. They are used as a pair to enable instrumentation of the whole root circumference. Many different sizes and shapes are available. Our preferred curettes are the Gracey 7/8 and the Columbia 13/14.

The procedure for *closed subgingival debridement* is as follows:

- The curette is inserted to the bottom of the gingival sulcus or pathological pocket

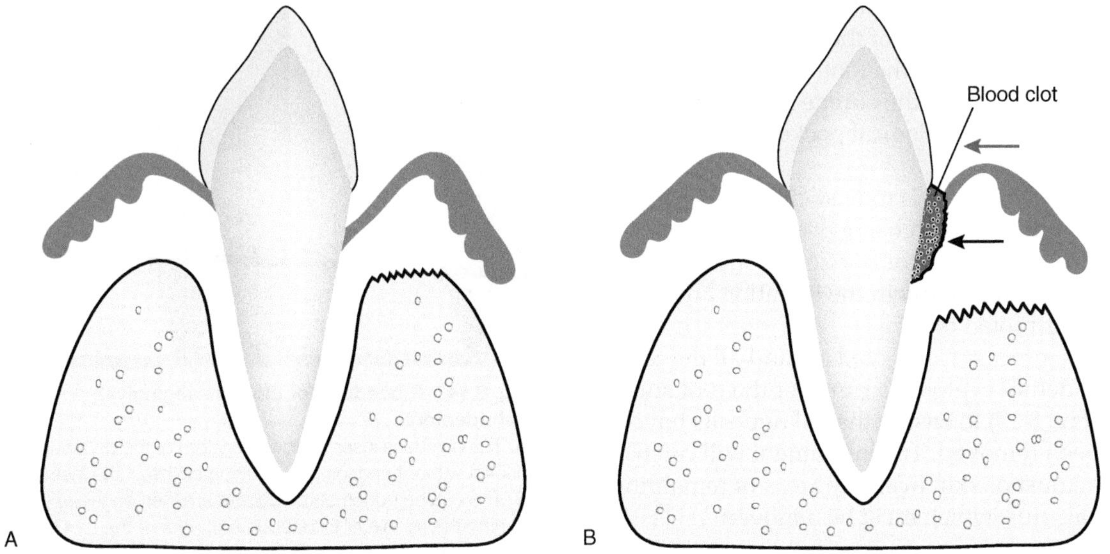

Fig. 8.13 Healing after subgingival debridement.
A: Before subgingival debridement.
B: Irrespective of whether a closed or open technique has been used for subgingival debridement, the epithelial attachment and pocket epithelium will have been removed during the procedure and a blood clot will have formed between the tooth and the connective tissue of the gingiva. As healing starts, both the epithelium and connective tissue are activated. The oral gingival epithelium will start to grow across to cover the exposed connective tissue (blue arrow) and the connective tissue starts to form new attachment with the clean root surface (black arrow).

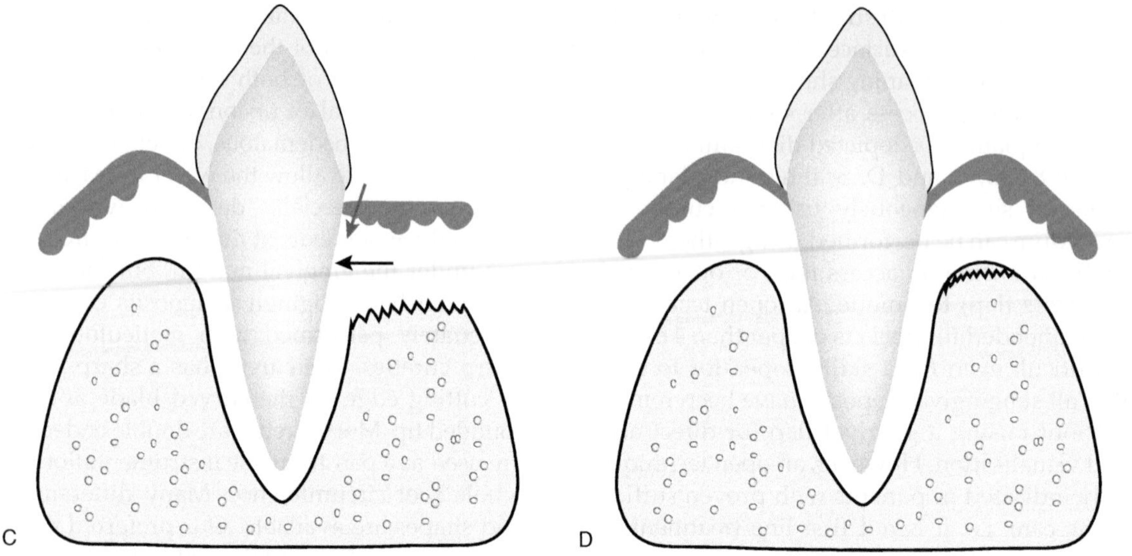

Fig. 8.13 Healing after subgingival debridement. *(contd)*
C: Once the oral epithelium has reached the tooth surface it will start to grow apically (blue arrow) and the situation becomes a race between the epithelium growing apically and the connective tissue attaching to the root surface (black arrow). The result of the race will determine at which level the epithelium's apical attachment will be.
D: The final stage of the healing process is the reformation of the normal epithelial attachment and gingival sulcus.

without engaging the cutting edges of the instrument (Fig. 8.14A)

- The cutting edges of the instrument are then engaged against the tooth root and sulcular epithelium and the curette is pulled out of the sulcus or pathological pocket in this position (Fig. 8.14B)
- The instrument is moved circumferentially around the tooth using overlapping vertical strokes. Oblique or horizontal strokes are also used, particularly in the furcation area of multirooted teeth
- The process is repeated around all the teeth
- A dental explorer is run over the root surface (Fig. 8.15) to ensure that all deposits have been removed. The instrument will catch against or skip over any areas of remaining calculus, which must be removed

A curette with two cutting edges will also remove the sulcular lining. Removing the inflamed sulcular epithelium is called subgingival curettage. It has been shown that subgingival curettage is not essential in controlling periodontal disease. The vital step is the removal of all subgingival

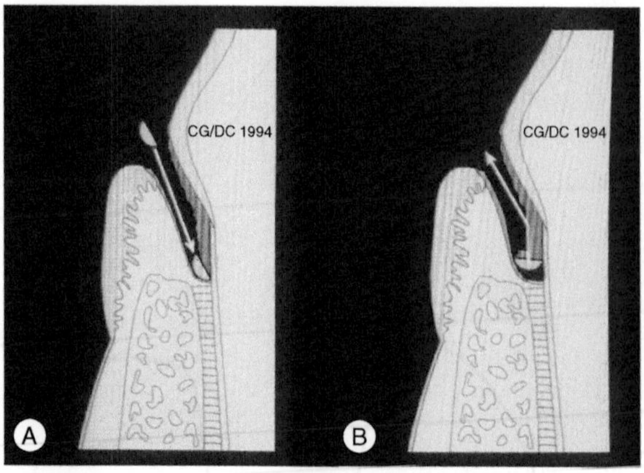

Fig. 8.14 Procedure for closed subgingival debridement.
A: The curette is inserted to the bottom of the periodontal pocket without engaging the cutting edges of the instrument.
B: The cutting edges of the curette are then engaged (by turning the handle of the instrument) against the root surface and pocket epithelium and the curette is pulled out of the pocket in this position. The instrument is worked in this way around the whole circumference of the tooth using overlapping strokes (mainly vertical, but oblique and horizontal strokes are also used, particularly in the furcation area of multirooted teeth).
(Reproduced from the *Manual of Small Animal Dentistry* with kind permission of BSAVA.)

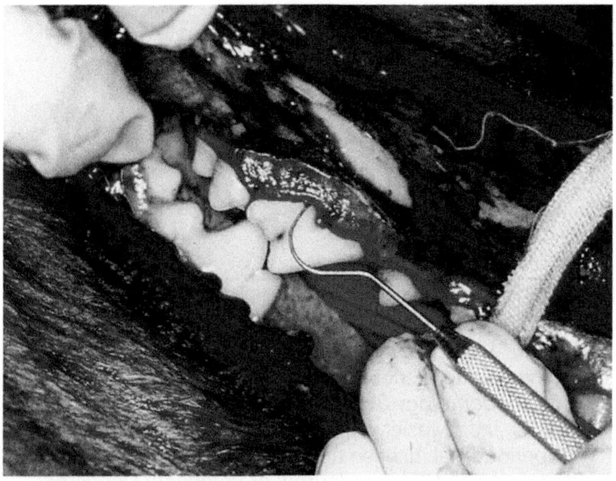

Fig. 8.15 Checking adequacy of subgingival debridement. A dental explorer is inserted below the gingival margin and run over the root surface to identify the presence of residual subgingival calculus, which needs to be removed.

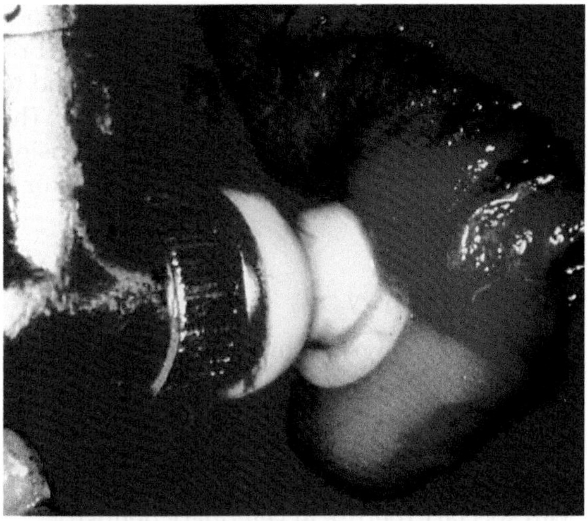

Fig. 8.16 Supragingival polishing. Polishing smoothes the tooth surface and helps remove any remaining plaque and stained pellicle. It is good practice to check the adequacy of the periodontal debriding by applying a plaque-disclosing solution after polishing. Any residual dental deposits can then be identified and removed.

deposits, i.e. subgingival scaling, and restoring the root surface to smoothness, i.e. root planing.

Subgingival debridement (scaling and root planing) takes time. A thorough procedure in an animal with extensive pocketing and subgingival deposits may well take an hour and often more. It must be emphasised that removing subgingival plaque, calculus and debris as well as the superficial layer of toxin-laden cementum and restoring the root surfaces to smoothness is a most important step. Removing only the supragingival debris at a periodontitis site does not have any therapeutic benefit. It will not prevent disease progression as the cause of the disease, namely subgingival plaque, is still present.

Polishing

Scaling, even when done correctly, will cause minor scratches of the tooth. A rough surface will facilitate plaque retention. Polishing smoothes this roughness and helps remove any remaining plaque and stained pellicle.

Polishing is best performed by applying a mildly abrasive prophylaxis paste to the tooth surface with a prophylaxis cup mounted in a slowly rotating low-speed handpiece. The handpiece should be running at less then 1000 rpm to avoid generating excessive heat by friction. The amount of heat which can easily result from incorrect polishing can cause severe pulpal pathology. A surplus of paste is applied to the tooth surface in a soft rubber cup using a light force, i.e. just enough force to cause the cup to flare out on the tooth surface. The prophylaxis cup is kept moving over the entire tooth surface for a few seconds per tooth. The flared edge of the prophylaxis cup can be used to polish slightly subgingivally, taking care to avoid causing any further gingival damage. This is illustrated in Figure 8.16. It is useful to check that all tooth surfaces are clean by using a plaque-disclosing solution after polishing. Any residual plaque is thus visualised and can be removed with further polishing.

It is not possible to polish the root surfaces within subgingival pockets (unless an open technique for subgingival debridement is used), so their smoothness must be assured by thorough, but not excessive, root planing.

Sulcular lavage

Sulcular lavage involves gently flushing the gingival sulcus and pathological pockets with saline or dilute chlorhexidine to remove any free-floating debris. This step is particularly important in a deep pathological pocket as free-floating debris may occlude the orifice of the pocket and lead to the formation of a lateral periodontal abscess. The stream of fluid is directed subgingivally using a blunt-ended needle, 'lachrymal' catheter or a Water Pik device.

Periodontal surgery

Periodontal surgery includes gingivectomy (gingivoplasty), various flap techniques (access flaps for open curettage, positioned flaps, etc.) and osseous surgery. Periodontal surgery is technically difficult and should be left to the veterinarian with special expertise in veterinary dentistry.

The main objective of periodontal surgery is to contribute to the preservation of the periodontium by facilitating plaque removal and plaque control. Periodontal surgery can help achieve this by;

1. Creating accessibility for professional scaling and root planing
2. Establishing a gingival morphology that facilitates plaque control by home care regimens.

Periodontal surgery is never first line treatment for periodontitis. Cause-related treatment, as described in this chapter, is always the first step in managing periodontitis. The effect of the cause-related therapy must be evaluated. If a client cannot maintain good dental hygiene for his pet then in the interest of the well-being of the animal there is no indication for periodontal surgery.

Summary

- The first bacteria to adhere to the pellicle are aerobic Gram-positive organisms
- The earliest sign of periodontal disease is gingivitis
- The primary cause of gingivitis and periodontitis is accumulation of dental plaque on the tooth surfaces
- In dogs and cats the main bacteria in supragingival plaque are *Actinomyces* and streptococci
- Dental calculus is mineralised plaque; its main importance in periodontal disease is as a plaque-retentive surface
- As plaque thickens, matures and extends further down the gingival sulcus, the environment becomes suitable for growth of anaerobic organisms, motile rods and spirochaetes
- The aim in periodontal disease prevention and treatment is to establish and maintain clinically healthy gingiva
- Radiography is mandatory if there is evidence of periodontitis disease clinically

REFERENCES

Allen, D.L. & Kerr, D.A. (1965) Tissue response in the guinea pig to sterile and non-sterile calculus. *Journal of Periodontology* **36**: 121–126.

DeBowes, L.J., Mosier, D., Logan, E. et al (1996) Association of periodontal disease and histologic lesions in multiple organs from 45 dogs. *Journal of Veterinary Dentistry* **13**(2): 57–60.

Egelberg, J. (1965) Local effects of diet on plaque formation and gingivitis development in dogs, 2. Effect of frequency of meals and tube feeding. *Odontolisk Revy* **16**: 50–60.

Engebretson, S.P., Lamster, I.B., Herrera-Abrev, M. et al (1999) The influence of interleukin gene polymorphism on expression of interleukin 1β and tumor necrosis factor-α in periodontal tissue and gingival crevicular fluid. *Journal of Periodontology* **70**: 567–573.

Hamp, S.E., Olsson, S.E., Farsø-Madsen, K. et al (1984) A macroscopic and radiologic investigation of dental diseases in dogs. *Veterinary Radiology* **25**: 86–92.

Hennet, P.R. & Harvey, C.E. (1991) Anaerobes in periodontal disease in the dog: a review. *Journal of Veterinary Dentistry* **8**(2): 18–21.

Kinane, D.F. & Lindhe, J. (1997) Pathogenesis of periodontitis. In: Lindhe, J., Karring, T. & Lang, N.P. (eds) *Clinical Periodontology and Implant Dentistry*. Copenhagen: Munksgaard, Ch. 5, pp. 189–225.

Kornman, K.S., Crane, A., Wang, H.Y. et al (1997) The interleukin 1 genotype as a severity factor in adult periodontal disease. *Journal of Clinical Periodontology* **24**(1): 72–77.

Listgarten, M.A. & Ellegaard, B. (1973) Electron microscopic evidence of a cellular attachment between junctional epithelium and dental calculus. *Journal of Periodontal Research* **8**: 143–150.

Löe, H., Theilade, E. & Jensen, S.B. (1965) Experimental gingivitis in man. *Journal of Periodontology* **36**: 177–187.

Loesche, W.J. (1979) Clinical and microbiological aspects of chemotherapeutic agents used according to the specific plaque hypothesis. *Journal of Dental Research* **58**: 2404–2414.

Love, D.N., Vekselstein, R. & Collings, S. (1990) The obligative and facultatively anaerobic bacterial flora of the normal feline gingival margin. *Veterinary Microbiology* **22**(2–3): 267–275.

Mallonee, D.H., Harvey, C.E., Venner, M. et al (1988) Bacteriology of periodontal disease in the cat. *Archives of Oral Biology* **33**(9): 677–683.

Mombelli, A., Nyman, S., Bragger, U. et al (1995) Clinical and microbiological changes associated with and altered subgingival environment induced by periodontal pocket reduction. *Journal of Clinical Periodontology* **22**(10): 780–787.

Nyman, S., Westfelt, E., Sarhes, G. et al (1988) Role of 'diseased' root cementum in healing following treatment of periodontal disease. A clinical study. *Journal of Clinical Periodontology* **15**(7): 464–468.

Nyman, S., Sarhed, G., Ericsson, I. et al (1986) Role of 'diseased' root cementum in healing following treatment of periodontal disease. An experimental study in the dog. *Journal of Periodontal Research* **21**(5): 496–503.

Reichart, P.A., Durr, U.M. & Triadan, H. (1984) Periodontal disease in the domestic cat: a histopathologic study. *Journal of Periodontal Research* **19**(1): 67–75.

Socransky, S.S., Haffajee, A.D., Smith, D.L. et al (1987) Difficulties encountered in the search for the etiologic agents of destructive periodontal disease. *Journal of Clinical Periodontology* **14**(10): 588–593.

Theilade, E. (1986) The non-specific theory in microbial etiology of inflammatory periodontal diseases. *Journal of Clinical Periodontology* **13**(10): 905–911.

Theilade, E., Wright, W.H., Jensen, S.B. et al (1966) Experimental gingivitis in man. II A longitudinal clinical and bacteriological investigation. *Journal of Periodontal Research* **1**: 1–13.

Thoden van Velzen, S.K., Abraham-Inpijn, L. & Moorer, W.R. (1984) Plaque and systemic disease: a reappraisal of the focal infection concept. *Journal of Clinical Periodontology* **11**(4): 209–220.

Waerhaug, J. (1956) Effect of rough surfaces upon gingival tissues. *Journal of Dental Research* **35**: 323–325.

9

Common oral and dental conditions

While the diagnosis of disease is the remit of the veterinarian, veterinary nurses and technicians need to be familiar with common oral and dental conditions to be able to identify them and record them on the dental chart. The details of oral and dental examination and recording are found in Chapter 6.

This chapter outlines common oral and dental conditions that are not covered elsewhere in this book. The clinical significance of the conditions and outline of treatment options are included for completeness. Some of the conditions may require no professional intervention; others can be managed successfully in the general practice (often by extraction) and some need referral to a specialist for treatment.

Periodontal disease is covered in Chapter 8. All dogs and cats require a combination of home care (daily toothbrushing and dental diet/dental hygiene chew) and professional cleaning. Preventive dentistry is indicated for every dog and cat and is detailed in Chapter 10. Dental conditions of lagomorphs and rodents are covered in Chapter 12.

DEVELOPMENTAL DENTAL DISORDERS

Developmental dental disorders may be due to abnormalities in the differentiation of the dental lamina and the tooth germs (anomalies in number, size and shape) or to abnormalities in the formation of the dental hard tissues (anomalies in structure).

Anomalies in number, size, and shape

Congenitally missing teeth

Congenital absence of teeth is common in the dog. Radiographs are required to determine if teeth missing on clinical examination are unerupted or actually absent (Fig. 9.1). This is often of interest for the owner of a dog meant for the show ring.

Absence of teeth can be an inherited abnormality or can result from disturbances during the initial stages of tooth formation. The primary teeth give rise to the permanent tooth buds, so if there is no primary tooth the permanent counterpart will also be missing. It is possible, however, for the primary tooth to be present and the permanent counterpart absent.

Total absence of teeth (anodontia) and congenital absence of many but not all teeth (oligodontia) are rare and can be associated with ectodermal dysplasia or occur in dogs with no apparent systemic problem or congenital syndrome (Andrews, 1972; Skrentary, 1964; Harvey & Emily, 1993). Absence of only a few teeth (hypodontia) is relatively common in dogs. It is especially common in purebred and line-bred dogs, as the genetic fault will have been perpetuated. It is also more common in small breed dogs. The premolars (Fig. 9.2) are the most commonly missing teeth (Harvey & Emily, 1993).

In general, missing teeth are of no clinical significance other than that plaque accumulation

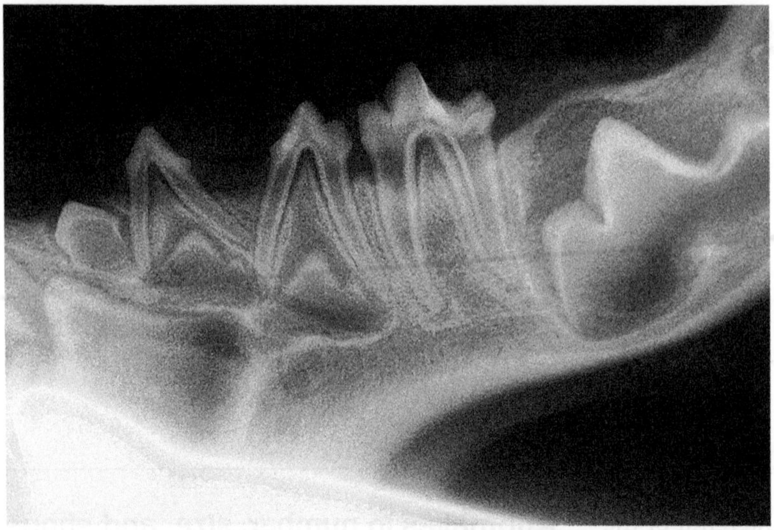

Fig. 9.1 Congenitally missing teeth. Radiographs are required to determine if teeth missing on clinical examination are unerupted or actually absent. This puppy has a missing permanent 4th premolar.

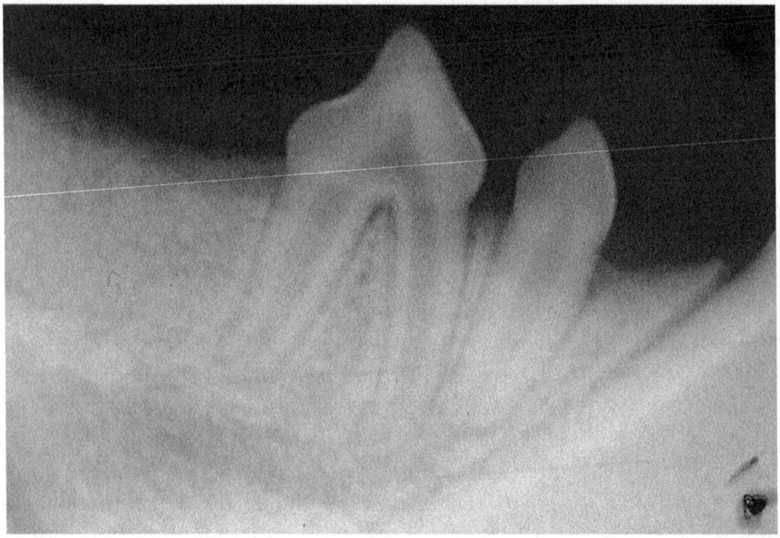

Fig. 9.2 Premolars are the most commonly missing teeth. The 3rd mandibular premolar was found to be missing on clinical examination. The radiograph shows that it is absent rather than unerupted.

may be more extensive as the cleaning of teeth associated with chewing is likely to be reduced.

Supernumerary teeth

Supernumerary teeth (Fig. 9.3) are common in certain dog breeds (Harvey & Emily, 1993). They are the result of either a genetic defect or a disturbance during tooth development. The duplication of teeth may affect the primary as well as the permanent dentition. Many supernumerary teeth resemble normal teeth, others have a conical shape, and some bear no resemblance to any normal tooth form. The most common complications caused by supernumerary teeth are malpositioning and non-eruption of other teeth (Harvey & Emily, 1993; Aitchison, 1963). As with other teeth that remain embedded, there is the possibility of cyst formation (Harvey & Emily, 1993; Shafer et al, 1974a; Stafne & Gibilisco, 1975a). Eruption and shedding disorders are covered later in this chapter. In addition, tooth crowding may contribute to

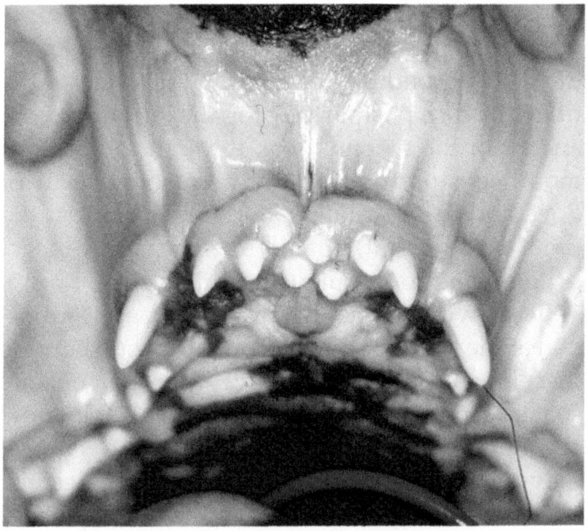

Fig. 9.3 Supernumerary teeth. Supernumerary teeth commonly cause crowding and malocclusion. Treatment consisted of extraction of the upper incisor teeth that were grossly out of alignment and had abnormal occlusion with the mandibular incisor teeth.

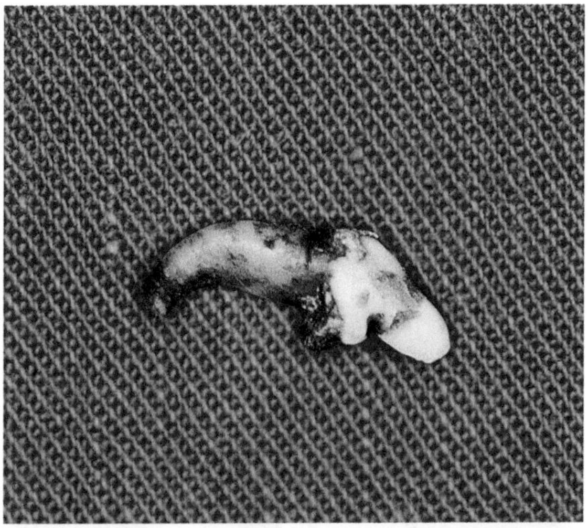

Fig. 9.4 Abnormalities in root shape. The upper 3rd incisor depicted has a marked curvature at its apex. Preoperative radiographs should be taken of all teeth where extraction is planned. Identification of an abnormality in root morphology allows selection of the optimal extraction technique. In this case, an open (surgical) extraction technique was chosen.

plaque accumulation and predispose to periodontal disease. Supernumerary teeth that contribute to malocclusion or crowding should be extracted (Harvey & Emily, 1993; Gorrel & Robinson, 1995). Radiographic evaluation allows differentiation between primary and permanent teeth. Primary teeth are smaller than their permanent counterparts; with long, slender roots. Compared with permanent teeth, the roots of primary teeth are relatively long in relation to the crown.

Fusion and gemination

Fusion is the developmental union of two or more teeth in which the dentine and one other dental tissue are united. There may be a complete union resulting in one abnormally large tooth, or union of the crowns, or union of the roots only. A supernumerary tooth is frequently one of the teeth involved. Gemination is an attempt to make two teeth from one enamel organ, without complete division. Fusion and gemination affect primary teeth as well as permanent ones.

If these teeth do not cause any functional problem, they do not need to be extracted.

Root abnormalities

Common root abnormalities include aberrations in shape (Fig. 9.4) and in the number of roots present (Fig. 9.5). They are not detected without radiographs. The identification of an abnormally shaped root or an extra root is not, in itself, an indication for treatment. However, if the tooth is affected by pathology that requires extraction, it is essential to have prior knowledge of an existing anatomical abnormality, so that the extraction can be planned accordingly (Fig. 9.6).

Anomalies in structure

Enamel hypoplasia (dysplasia)

Enamel hypoplasia (dysplasia) may be defined as an incomplete or defective formation of the organic enamel matrix of teeth. The result is defective (soft, porous) enamel. It can be caused by local, systemic or hereditary factors. Depending on the cause, the condition can affect one or only a few teeth (localised form), or all teeth in the dentition (generalised form). It is essential to remember that enamel hypoplasia results only if the injury occurs during the formative stage of enamel development, i.e. during amelogenesis.

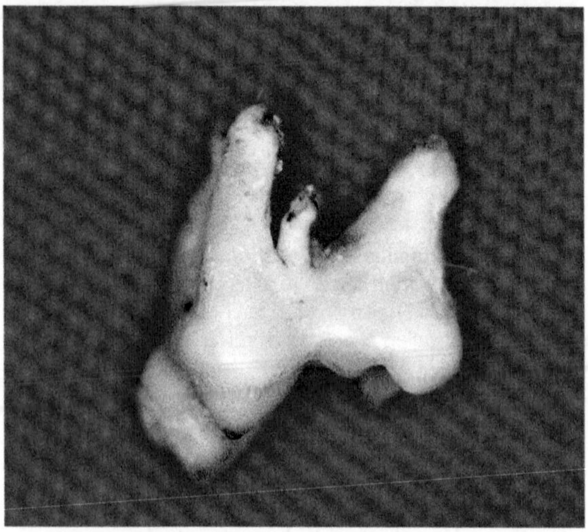

Fig. 9.5 Abnormalities in the number of roots. The upper 1st molar depicted has a small extra root. It was identified on preoperative radiographs. The tooth was extracted due to severe periodontitis and could thus be removed without prior sectioning into single-rooted segments.

Thus, the defect occurs before the tooth erupts into the oral cavity. Crown formation lasts from the forty-second day of gestation through to the fifteenth day postpartum for the primary teeth and from the second week through to the third month postpartum for the permanent teeth of dogs and cats (Arnall, 1960). Depending on the time of the insult, enamel dysplasia will affect primary and/or permanent teeth.

Teeth with enamel dysplasia may appear normal at the time of eruption, but they soon become discoloured as the defective (porous) enamel soaks up pigments (from food, soil, etc.). In more severely affected teeth, the defective enamel may flake off with use. In very severe cases, the enamel is visibly deficient, discoloured in patches or partly missing already at the time of eruption.

If the enamel dysplasia is the result of a local trauma (Fig. 9.7A) or systemic pyrexia (Fig. 9.8A) that resolves within a period of time, only those areas undergoing active formation during the period of the insult will be affected. This is seen clinically as bands of dysplastic enamel encircling the crown, with areas of normal enamel elsewhere on the tooth. Banding is evident in Figures 9.7A and 9.8A.

Poorly protected or exposed dentine is painful. These teeth do become less sensitive with increasing age of the animal since secondary

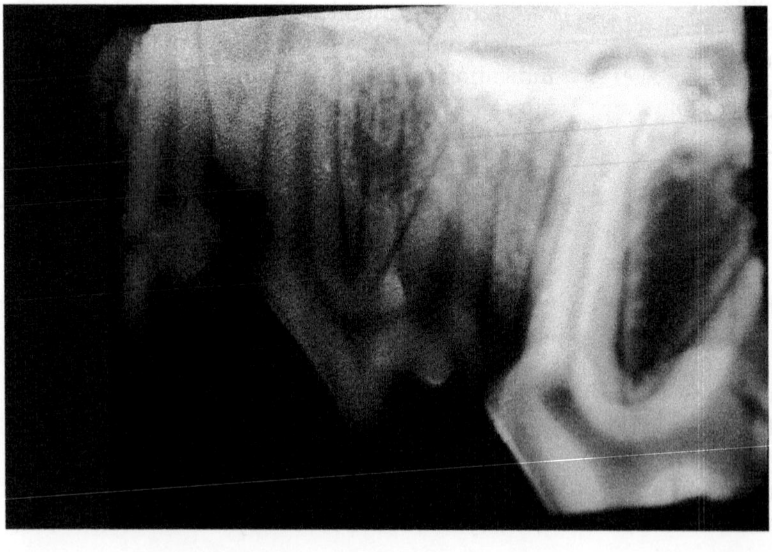

Fig. 9.6 Abnormalities in the number of roots. The maxillary 3rd premolar depicted on the radiograph has a palatal root, as well as the expected mesial and distal roots. This was an incidental finding on full mouth radiographs. It was bilateral, i.e. both left and right maxillary 3rd premolars had an extra palatal root. If this tooth were to require extraction, it would need to be sectioned into three single-rooted segments rather than the usual two single-rooted segments.

dentine is laid down continuously by the pulp. Another consideration is that dysplastic enamel harbours dental plaque. In severe cases of generalised enamel hypoplasia, where the dentine is effectively exposed to the oral environment, chronic pulp disease and potentially periapical disease may occur due to pulpal irritation via the poorly protected or exposed dentine tubules (Fig. 9.8B). Pulp and periapical pathology is detailed later in the chapter. Teeth affected by such pathology require treatment, i.e. either extraction or referral to a specialist for endodontic therapy (outlined in Appendix 2), if they are to be maintained.

In the management of patients affected by enamel dysplasia, oral hygiene is of paramount importance. Daily plaque removal will promote periodontal health and possibly reduce pulpal irritation. Affected animals require radiographic assessment and monitoring to detect complications such as pulp and periapical disease. In fact, a series of full mouth radiographs at regular intervals is indicated. In young animals exhibiting signs of discomfort, topical fluoride application may be beneficial. Topical fluoride application will enhance enamel remineralisation and 'harden' the enamel. It must be remembered that fluoride is potentially toxic and the risk of systemic administration of fluoride products meant for topical application is greater in the dog and cat as they will swallow these products (Gorrel, 2003). The use of professionally applied varnishes and

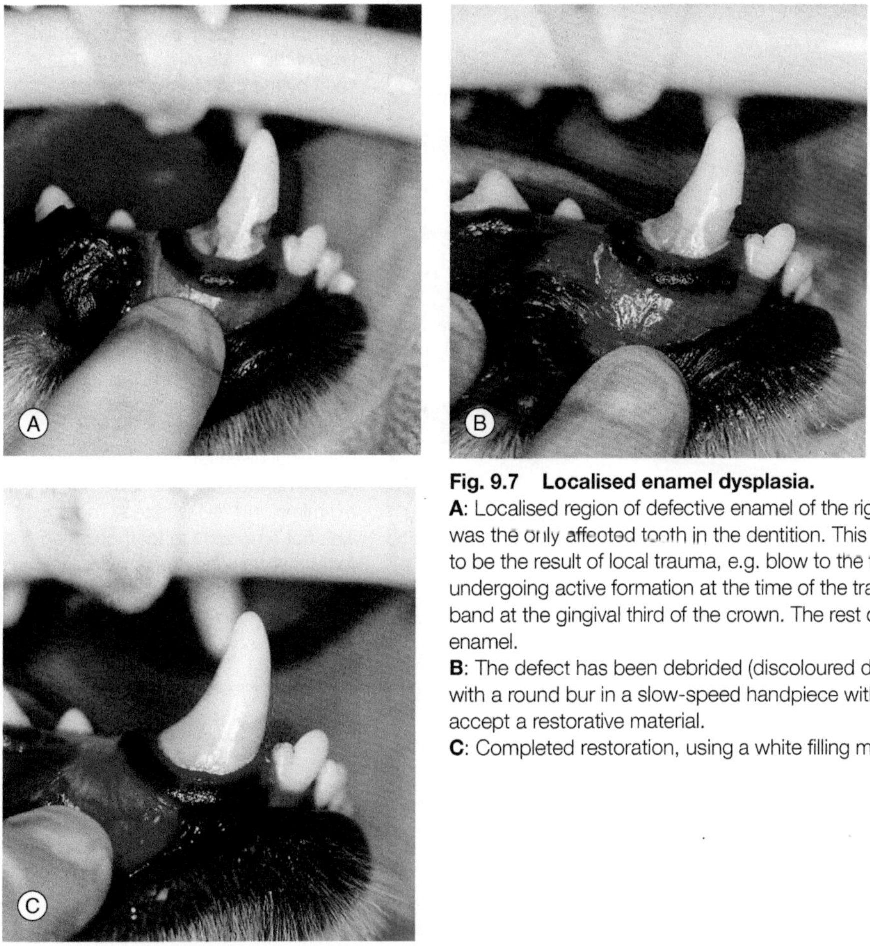

Fig. 9.7 Localised enamel dysplasia.
A: Localised region of defective enamel of the right mandibular canine tooth. This was the only affected tooth in the dentition. This type of enamel dysplasia is likely to be the result of local trauma, e.g. blow to the face. Only the region of enamel undergoing active formation at the time of the trauma is defective, appearing as a band at the gingival third of the crown. The rest of the crown is covered by normal enamel.
B: The defect has been debrided (discoloured dysplastic enamel was removed with a round bur in a slow-speed handpiece with water cooling) and prepared to accept a restorative material.
C: Completed restoration, using a white filling material.

gels associated with a moderate rise in plasma fluoride concentrations may well be safer than daily use of fluoride-containing toothpastes (Gorrel, 2003). In other words, it is useful to apply fluoride varnishes or gel at regular intervals. The best way to do this is following a dental cleaning. The product is applied while the animal is under general anaesthesia and excess is removed before the animal is allowed to recover. In severely affected cases, the enamel is so soft that it is removed on scaling. In these patients, gross calculus accumulation is carefully removed with hand instruments (a scaler or curette) rather than powered scalers (sonic or ultrasonic). The crowns are polished with a fine grain (to reduce abrasion) prophy paste. Restoration of lost enamel, i.e. debriding the defect and replacing lost tissue with a suitable filling material, is useful for smaller lesions (Fig. 9.7B, C) as it protects against dentine sensitivity. It is not practical for extensive, generalised lesions. Restoration requires referral to a specialist.

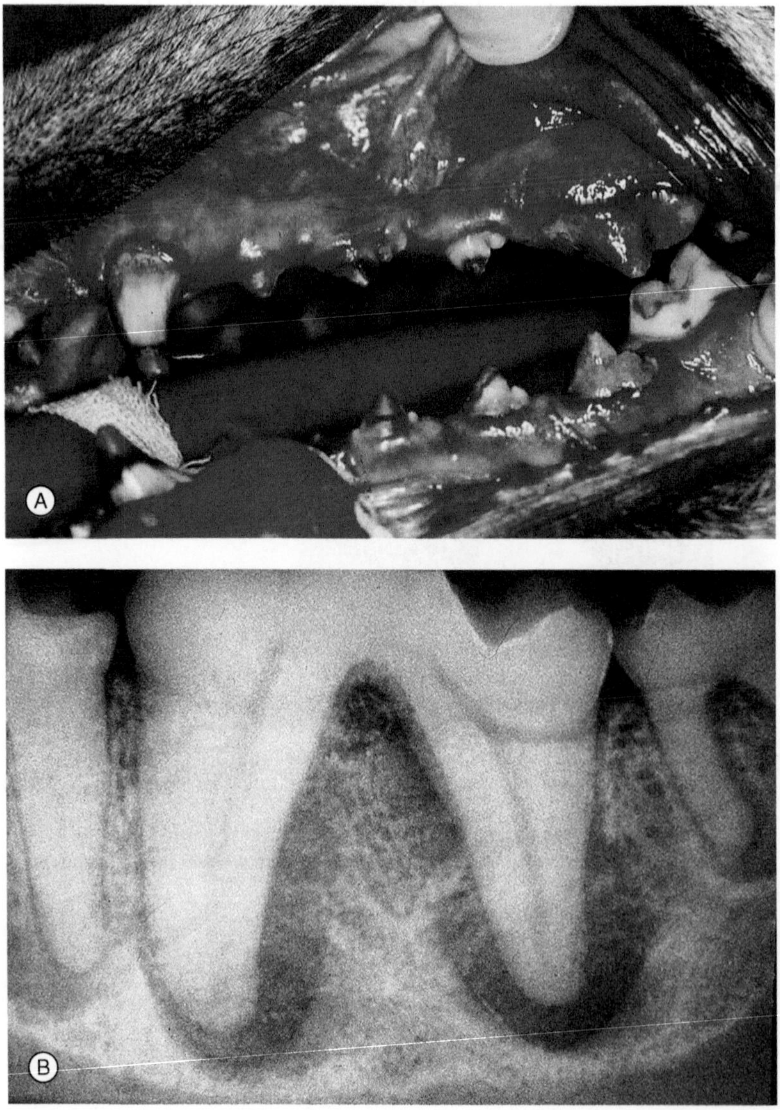

Fig. 9.8 Generalised enamel dysplasia.
A: Enamel dysplasia affecting all teeth of the dentition. This type of enamel dysplasia is likely to be caused by systemic factors, e.g. pyrexia, at the time of active enamel development. Only the areas actively forming at the time of the insult will be affected as is seen by the obvious banding with areas of normal enamel elsewhere on the tooth.
B: Radiograph of the caudal left mandible of the same dog reveals pulp and periapical disease affecting the mandibular 4th premolar and the 1st and 2nd molars. The full mouth radiographic series showed that almost all teeth of the dentition had evidence of pulp and periapical pathology. Treatment consisted of extraction of all teeth except the incisors and canines (as these were unaffected by pulp and periapical disease). Home care was recommended and annual radiographic examination was instituted. The dog was not amenable to toothbrushing and further extractions due to pulp and periapical pathology have been performed.

DISORDERS OF ERUPTION AND SHEDDING

Unerupted teeth can be detected and evaluated by radiographic examination only (Fig. 9.9). Embedded teeth are those that have failed to erupt and remain completely or partially covered by bone or soft tissue or both. Those that have been obstructed by contact against another erupted or non-erupted tooth in the course of their eruption are referred to as impacted teeth (Stafne & Gibilisco, 1975b).

The causes for non-eruption of teeth are numerous (Andrews, 1972; Stafne & Gibilisco, 1975b). In humans, the most common cause is lack of space. Another common cause is obstruction, either by persistent (retained beyond their normal time for exfoliation) primary teeth or by supernumerary teeth. In the dog, persistent primary teeth more commonly result in abnormal positioning of the permanent tooth rather than non-eruption (Harvey & Emily, 1993). Consequently, persistent primary teeth should be extracted. Cyst and tumours may also obstruct eruption of the teeth. Other possible causes for non-eruption of teeth include infection; trauma; anomalous conditions affecting the jaws and teeth, e.g. abnormal primary displacement of the tooth bud; and systemic conditions which cause underdevelopment of the jaws, structural defects of the teeth, or poor quality of bone.

Unerupted teeth may cause no pathology, in which case they do not require any treatment. If an obstruction to eruption can be clearly identified, e.g. supernumerary tooth, it should be removed. An increased risk of cyst formation has been reported with unerupted teeth (Stafne & Gibilisco, 1975a). The follicle of the unerupted tooth undergoes cystic transformation. Follicular (dentigerous) cysts can become large and cause extensive resorption of the surrounding alveolar bone. Consequently, unerupted teeth that are maintained require regular radiographic monitoring to identify development of a follicular cyst at an early stage. Treatment then consists of removing the unerupted tooth and its associated cyst. Some veterinarians choose to extract unerupted teeth as a prophylactic measure.

WEAR OF DENTAL HARD TISSUE

Attrition is the loss of tooth substance that results from wear that is produced by opposing teeth coming into contact with one another, i.e. teeth that have occlusal contact. Attrition is therefore also called occlusal wear. Incisal wear is the term used when describing attrition of the incisor

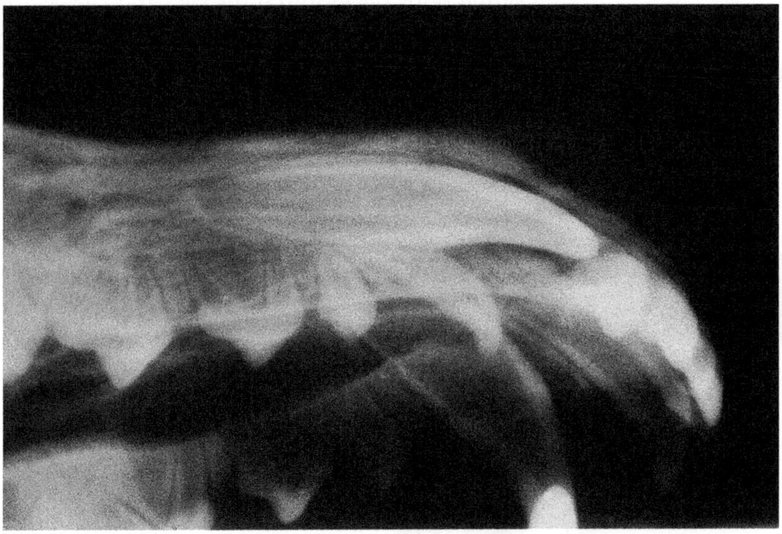

Fig. 9.9 Unerupted teeth. Unerupted teeth can only be detected and evaluated by radiographic examination. In this patient, the right permanent maxillary canine tooth has not erupted and the right primary maxillary canine tooth is persistent. The owner was not amenable to the regular radiographic evaluation required if the unerupted permanent tooth were to be maintained. The chosen treatment in this case therefore consisted of extracting (open/surgical technique) both the persistent primary canine and the unerupted permanent canine.

region. There is progressive attrition with increasing age, resulting in the wearing away of the cusps and exposure of the dentine (Fig. 9.10). The deposition of reparative dentine keeps pace with the loss of tooth substance and there is rarely pulpal exposure. In fact, the crown pulp may come close to obliteration. In other words, attrition is a physiological event that occurs, to varying degrees, in all individuals. Factors such as loss of teeth, malocclusion and habits such as stone chewing may produce excessive attrition, i.e. attrition that is so rapid that the formation of reparative dentine cannot keep pace with it, and pulp exposure results (Stafne & Gibilisco, 1975c).

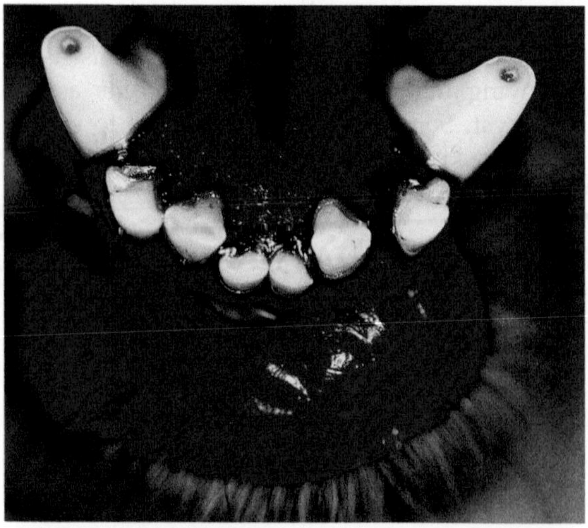

Fig. 9.10 Wear of dental tissue. As the enamel is worn away, the dentine is exposed to the oral environment. The deposition of reparative dentine keeps pace with the loss of tooth substance and there is rarely pulpal exposure. The exposed dentine is yellow to brown and has a hard surface on exploration with a dental probe/explorer.

Abrasion is the wearing away of tooth structure which is not caused by incisal or occlusal wear. In other words, wear of tooth surfaces that are not in contact. In humans, the most common cause of abrasion is incorrect use of a toothbrush, resulting in abrasion of the buccal tooth surfaces, usually just above the gingival margin. In the dog, the most common cause of abrasion is cage biting. The hard tissues on the distal aspect of the maxillary canine teeth are progressively lost, weakening the tooth, until the crown fractures (generally with pulpal exposure).

The consequences of pulpal exposure, whether caused by excessive attrition or abrasion, are detailed later in the chapter. An exposed pulp always requires treatment, either by extraction of the affected tooth or endodontic therapy, which allows the tooth to be maintained. Measures to prevent excessive attrition and abrasion should be instituted. These are detailed in Chapter 10.

CARIES

Caries (dental decay) occurs in dogs. In our experience, medium and large breed dogs are more commonly affected and the lesions usually affect the teeth that have true occlusal tables, namely the molar teeth (Fig. 9.11). Caries has not been described in cats.

While both periodontal disease and caries are caused by the accumulation of dental plaque on the tooth surfaces, the pathogenesis of the two diseases is completely different. Periodontal

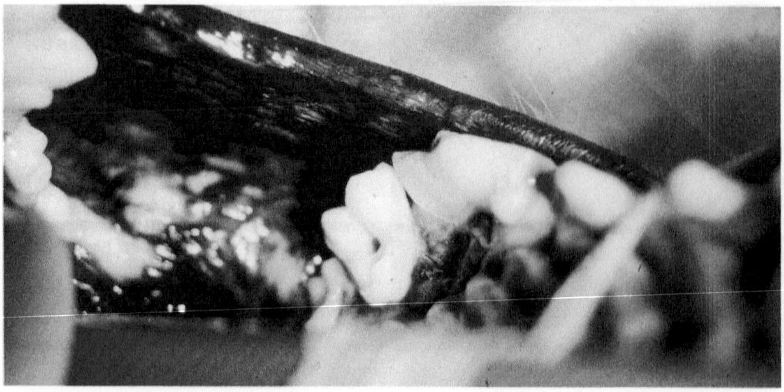

Fig. 9.11 Occlusal caries. Dental caries usually affects the tooth surfaces that have true occlusal tables, namely the molars. The discoloured, soft (an explorer 'catches' in the tooth surface) area in the centre of the occlusal table of the maxillary 1st molar is occlusal caries. All occlusal surfaces, whether discoloured or not, should be meticulously examined with a sharp dental explorer.

disease is a plaque-induced inflammation of the periodontium and caries is a plaque-induced destruction of the hard tissues of the tooth. Caries starts as an inorganic demineralisation of the enamel. The demineralisation occurs when plaque bacteria use fermentable carbohydrate (notably sugar) from the diet as a source of energy. The fermentation products are acidic and demineralise the enamel. Once the enamel has been destroyed, the process extends into the dentine. In the dentine, the process accelerates as an organic decay and will eventually involve the pulp, causing pulpitis and possibly pulp necrosis and/or periapical pathology. Dental caries stimulates the formation of reparative dentine on the surface of the pulpal wall, which is directly beneath it (Stafne & Gibilisco, 1975c, 1975d; Shafer et al, 1974b, 1974c). If the carious lesion is progressing slowly, the deposition of reparative dentine may keep pace with its advance and prevent exposure of the dental pulp.

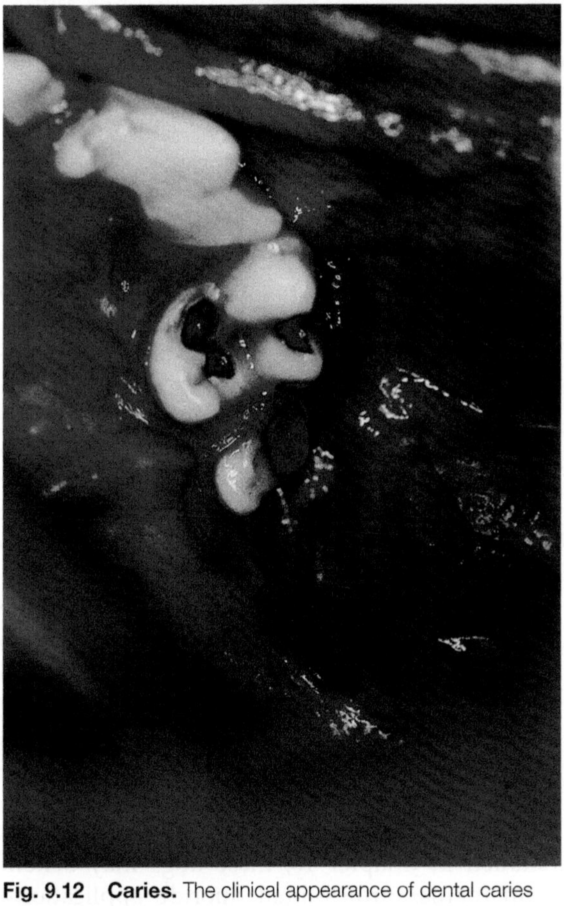

Fig. 9.12 Caries. The clinical appearance of dental caries affecting the left 1st and 2nd molars is depicted. The black areas were soft on exploration, with the explorer readily 'catching' in the tooth surface. Radiographs are indicated to assess the full extent of the lesions and select appropriate treatment, i.e. extraction or referral.

The initial inorganic demineralisation can be halted as long as the process has not reached the enamel–dentine junction. Meticulous dental hygiene in combination with topical fluoride treatment and dietary restrictions (reducing the frequency of intake of easily fermentable carbohydrate) can lead to remineralisation of the initial defect. An enamel 'scar' will, however, always be present (Stafne & Gibilisco, 1975c; Shafer et al, 1974b). However, if the process has entered the dentine it becomes irreversible and progressive. Treatment (restoration or extraction) becomes mandatory. In the dog, caries is very rarely diagnosed at the early enamel demineralisation stage. It is usually diagnosed only when the process already involves the dentine (Fig. 9.12) or the pulp is exposed (Figs 9.13 and 9.14). The reason why caries is rarely diagnosed at the enamel

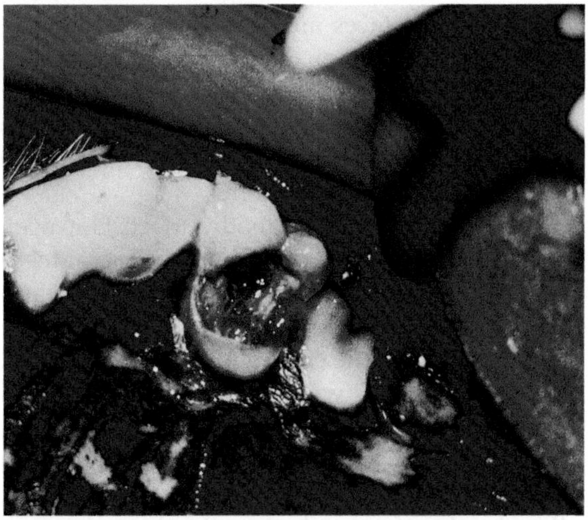

Fig. 9.13 Extensive caries. The carious lesion of the maxillary 1st molar depicted here has resulted in extensive loss of enamel and dentine and exposed the pulp chamber to the oral cavity. The pink tissue seen in the centre of the occlusal table is inflamed and hyperplastic pulp tissue (pulp granuloma). Radiographs reveal that the dentine destruction has been so extensive that the furcation of the roots has been broached, i.e. the three roots are unconnected to the crown. Extraction is the only treatment possible for this tooth!

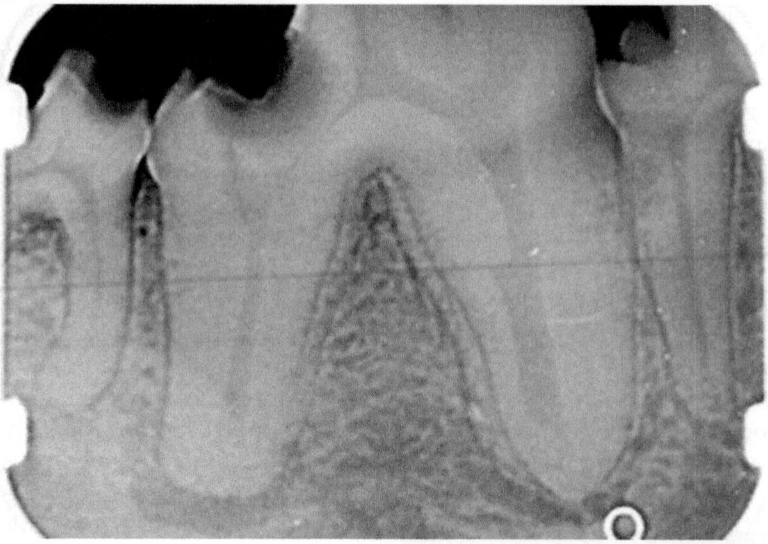

Fig. 9.14 Radiograph of a tooth with an extensive carious lesion. The radiograph of the right mandibular 1st molar shows an extensive carious lesion on the distal occlusal surface. The process extends into the root pulp. Periapical lesions of both roots are obvious. Treatment consists of extraction or referral for endodontic therapy and restoration.

demineralisation stage in dogs is twofold. First, the occlusal surfaces are not generally explored with a sharp explorer during clinical examination. Moreover, dog enamel is comparatively thinner than human enamel and the process is thus likely to extend into the dentine more rapidly than in human patients.

Caries can occur on any tooth surface. However, the occlusal (grinding) surfaces of the molar teeth seem predisposed in dogs. Clinically, caries manifests as softened, often discoloured (dark brown or black spots) in the enamel (Figs 9.11 and 9.12). A dental explorer will 'catch' in the softened carious tooth surface. A small enamel defect covers a large cavern of decayed dentine. Note that not all lesions are grossly discoloured and all occlusal surfaces, whether discoloured or not, should be meticulously examined with a dental explorer. If the explorer sticks in the tooth surface, then caries should be suspected and radiographs are indicated. Radiographically, radiolucent defects are seen in the affected area of the crown. Radiographs will also give an indication of how close to the pulp chamber a caries lesion extends (the extent of reparative dentine formation and the amount and thickness of dentine that separates the pulp from the carious lesion), which allows selection of the most appropriate treatment. Discoloured areas that are hard and in which the explorer does not 'catch' are not caries. They could be exposed dentine due to attrition or stain.

Diagnosed caries requires treatment. The options are extraction or referral to a specialist for restoration (if the process involves the pulp tissue as in Fig. 9.14, endodontic therapy prior to restoration is required). If the process has resulted in gross loss of tooth substance at the time of diagnosis, then extraction is the only option (Fig. 9.13). Measures to prevent new lesions must be instituted in animals with diagnosed caries. In addition to home care and dietary modifications as detailed in Chapter 10, these dogs may benefit from regular professional fluoride applications. Fluoride enhances remineralisation and makes the enamel more resistant to the acid dissolution that occurs with caries.

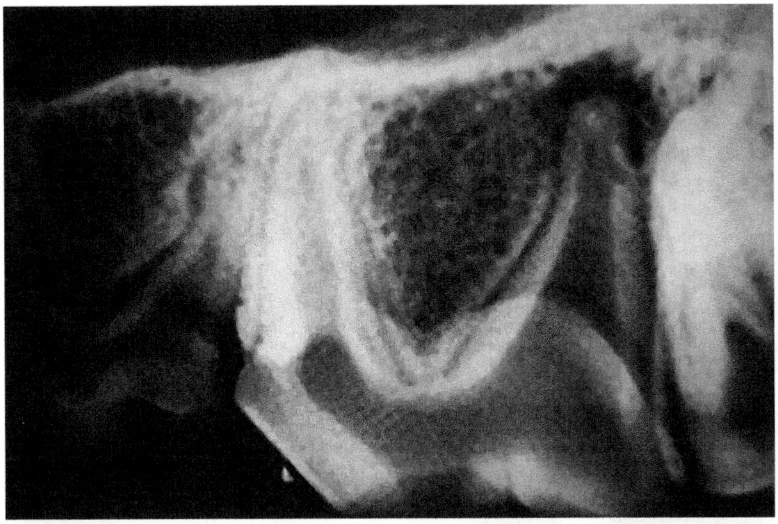

Fig. 9.15 Periapical pathology. Destruction of the bone surrounding the apex of the tooth is evident as rarefaction on a radiograph. In the radiograph depicted, there is an obvious periapical lesion of the distal root of the left maxillary 4th premolar. This tooth requires referral for endodontic therapy if it is to be maintained. Extraction is the other option.

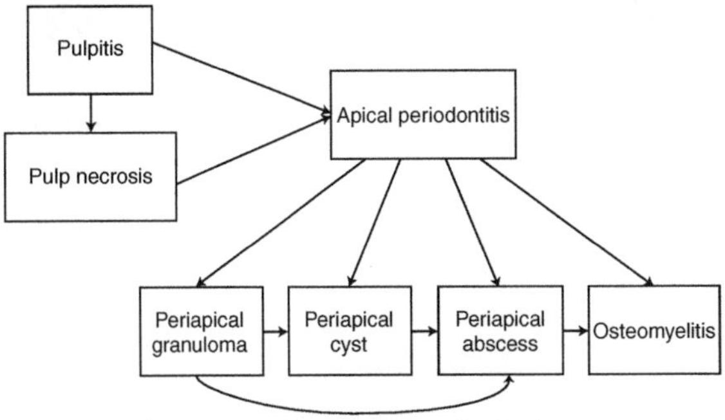

Fig. 9.16 Summary of pulp and periapical pathophysiology.

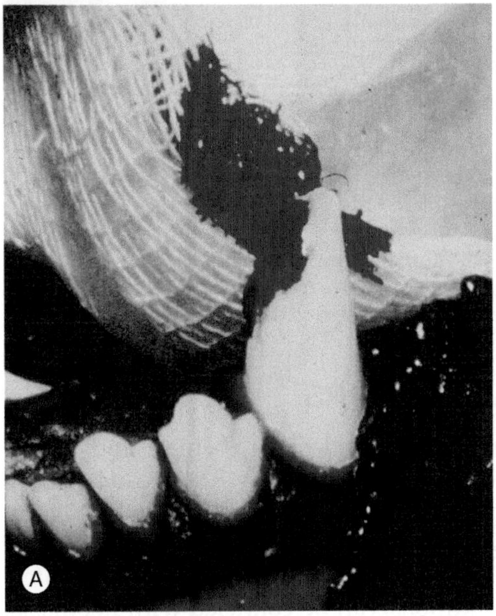

Fig. 9.17 Tooth fracture.
A: Fresh (trauma occurred 15 minutes earlier) crown fracture with an exposed and bleeding pulp.

PULP AND PERIAPICAL DISEASES

Insults (e.g. heat, infarction, bacteria, mechanical trauma) to the pulp of a tooth will result in inflammation, i.e. pulpitis. Untreated pulpitis will ultimately result in pulp necrosis. The term periapical disease is used to include inflammatory lesions resulting in destruction of the apical periodontium and bone around the apex of the tooth (Fig. 9.15). Periapical pathology occurs as an extension of untreated pulpal disease (Fig. 9.16).

In dogs and cats, pulp and consequent periapical diseases are common and are usually a sequel to traumatic tooth injures, either tooth fracture (Fig. 9.17 A, B and C) or damage to the periodontium. They are generally the result of a road traffic accident, blunt blow to the face, or chewing on hard objects. A tooth affected by pulp and periapical diseases should always be treated, i.e. it cannot just be ignored. In general terms, treatment is either extraction or endodontic therapy. The principles of endodontic therapy, which allows a tooth to be maintained, are outlined in Appendix 2.

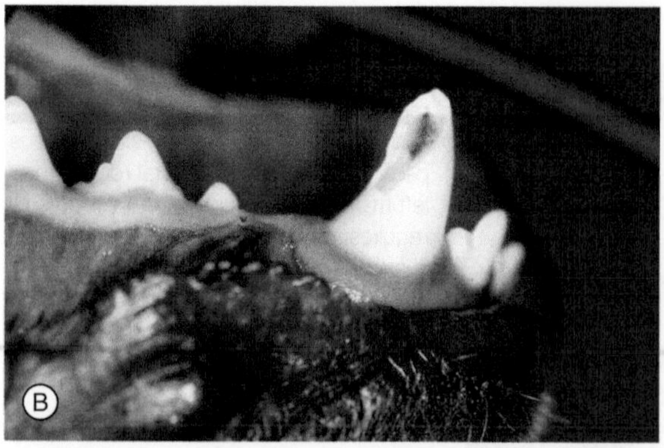

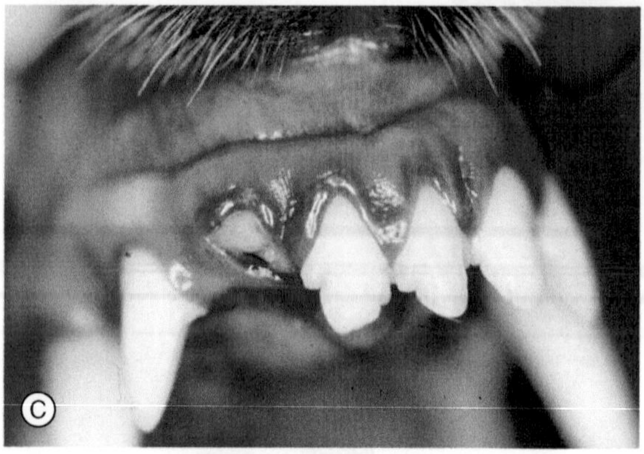

Fig. 9.17 Tooth fracture. *(contd)*
B: Crown fracture with an exposed and inflamed pulp.
C: Crown fracture with an exposed and necrotic pulp.

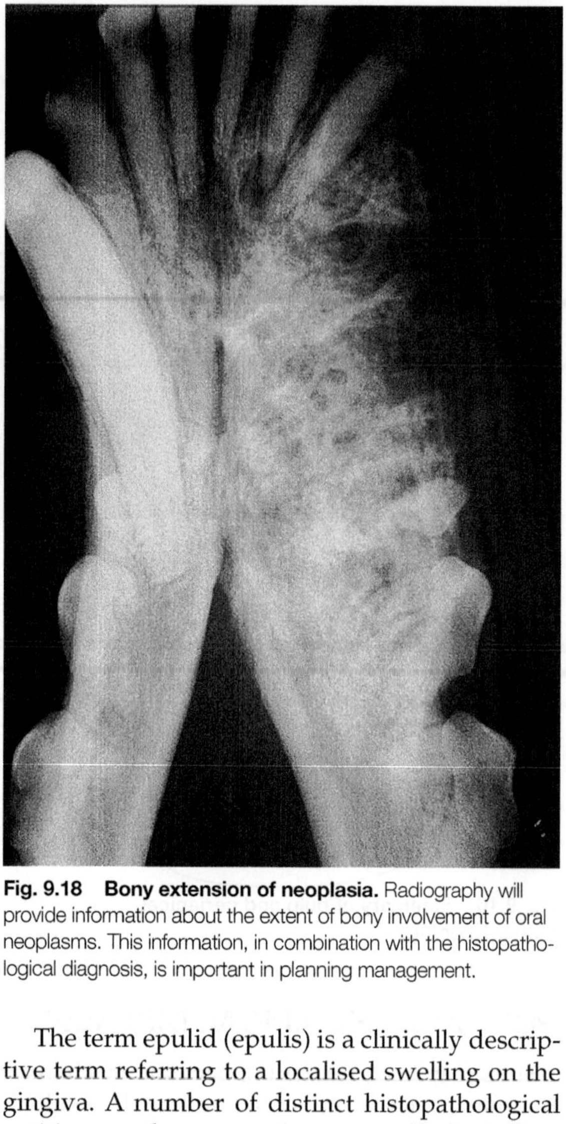

Fig. 9.18 Bony extension of neoplasia. Radiography will provide information about the extent of bony involvement of oral neoplasms. This information, in combination with the histopathological diagnosis, is important in planning management.

ORAL TUMOURS

Various neoplastic lesions (benign and malignant) occur in the oral cavity. These can be odontogenic (from dental tissue) or non-odontogenic in origin. In addition, non-neoplastic lesions and swellings, e.g. gingival hyperplasia and infective conditions, can be confused with neoplasia. Conversely, oral neoplasms may present as non-healing ulcerative lesions rather than as masses. In addition, the so-called epulides constitute a variety of pathological entities.

Malignant neoplasm of the mouth and pharynx constitute 5–7% of all canine tumours (Verstraete, 1995). The most common malignant neoplasms are malignant melanoma (30–35%), squamous cell carcinoma (20–30%) and fibrosarcoma (1–20%) (Verstraete, 1995). Osteosarcoma is also relatively common.

The term epulid (epulis) is a clinically descriptive term referring to a localised swelling on the gingiva. A number of distinct histopathological entities can thus present as an epulis, including malignant tumours. However, most epulides are non-neoplastic lesions or odontogenic tumours. In a recent study (Verstraete et al, 1992), it was found that 44% of epulides were focal fibrous hyperplasia. Peripheral odontogenic fibromas were also common (17%) and peripheral ameloblastoma accounted for 18% of epulides examined histologically.

Radiography while not diagnostic of the tumour type will provide information about the extent of bony involvement of oral neoplasms (Fig. 9.18). Such information, in conjunction with the histopathological diagnosis, is important in planning tumour management.

ROOT RESORPTION

Hard tissues are protected from resorption by their surface layer of cells (Gunnraj, 1999; Lindskog & Hammarström, 1980). Internal root resorption (when the root is resorbing from the pulp side towards the external tooth surface) is triggered by pulpal inflammation. External root resorption (when the root is resorbing from the cementum towards the pulp) may follow any damage to the protective periodontal ligament and cementoblast layer. Inflammatory external root resorption is seen as a complication to orthodontic treatment, in periodontitis and in conjunction with periapical pathology.

External root resorption (odontoclastic resorptive lesions) of unknown aetiology is common in cats. This type of idiopathic tooth resorption has also been shown to occur in feral (Clarke & Cameron, 1997; Verstraete et al, 1996) and wild cats (Levin, 1996; Berger et al, 1996). They have also been reported in the dog (Arnbjerg, 1996) and in the chinchilla (Crossley et al, 1997).

Odontoclastic resorptive lesions (ORL) are a type of 'idiopathic' external root resorption, where the hard tissues of the root surfaces are destroyed by the activity of multinucleated cells called odontoclasts. The destroyed root surface is replaced by cementum- or bone-like tissue. The process (Fig. 9.19 A, B and C) starts in cementum and progresses to involve the dentine, where it spreads along the dentine tubules and eventually comes to involve the dentine of the crown as well as the root. The peri-pulpal dentine is relatively resistant to resorption and the pulp thus only becomes involved late in the disease. The process extends through the crown dentine, eventually reaching the enamel. The enamel is either resorbed or it fractures off and a cavity becomes clinically evident (Figs 9.20 and 9.21A). In the absence of routine radiography, the lesions are first noted clinically when they become evident in the crown, often as cavities at the cemento-enamel junction (CEJ). Figure 9.21B depicts the radiographic appearance of the clinical lesion

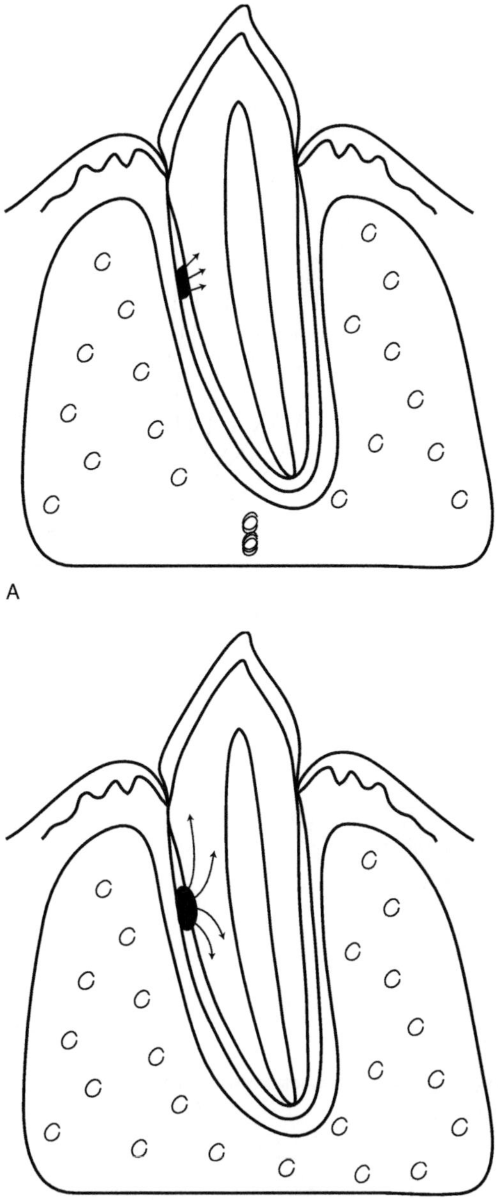

A

B

Fig. 9.19 Development of ORL.
A: The process starts anywhere on the root surface.
B: Once cementum has been destroyed, the process extends into the dentine and spreads apically and coronally.

seen in Figure 9.21A. The first clinical manifestation of ORL is thus a late-stage lesion. In many cases, the progressive dentine destruction with ORL, weakens and undermines the crown to such an extent that minor trauma, e.g. during

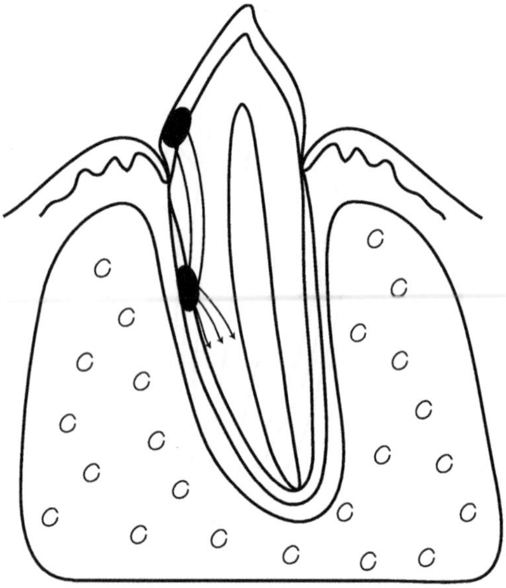

Fig. 9.19 Development of ORL. *(contd)*
C: The process extends through the crown dentine, eventually reaching the enamel, which is either resorbed or fractures off and a cavity becomes clinically evident.

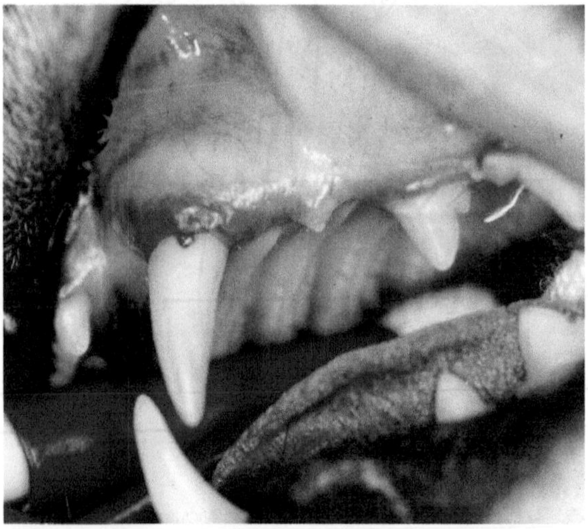

Fig. 9.20 Clinical appearance of ORL. The lesions are first noticed clinically when they become evident in the crown, often as a cavity at the CEJ. The process has extended into the crown dentine and come to involve the enamel, which has either resorbed or fractured off to reveal a small cavity, filled with granulation-like tissue, at the buccal aspect of the gingival margin of the upper canine. Contrary to common belief, this is a late-stage lesion.

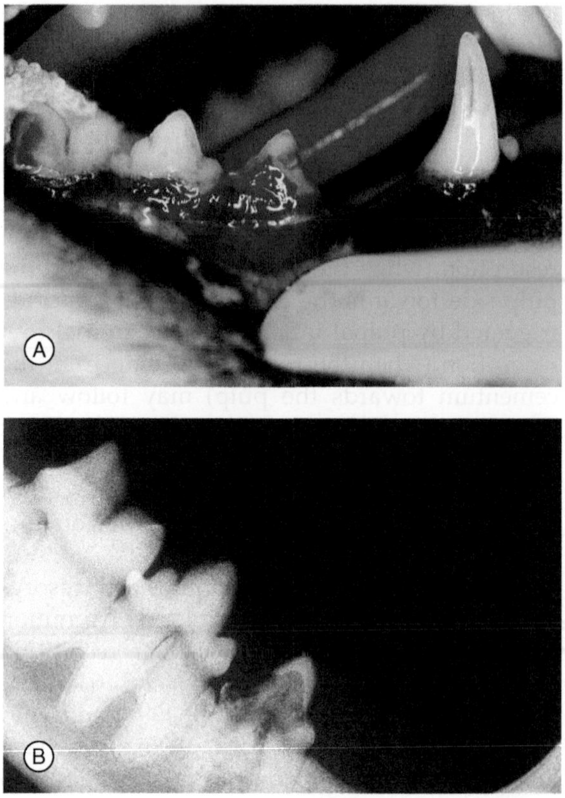

Fig. 9.21 Clinical and radiographic appearance of ORL.
A: Clinical appearance. The lower left 3rd premolar tooth has an extensive cavity at the CEJ. The destroyed dentine and enamel have been replaced by connective tissue. Again, this is a late-stage lesion.
B: The radiographic appearance of the left 3rd mandibular premolar tooth depicted in A. Both roots show evidence of extensive resorption, i.e. loss of distinct periodontal ligament space, replacement of tooth substance by bone-like material, and most of the crown dentine is destroyed. This tooth requires treatment.

chewing, causes the crown to fracture off, leaving the root in the alveolar bone. The resorbing root remnants are usually covered by intact gingiva (Fig. 9.22 A, B). However, in some cases the overlying gingiva may be inflamed (Fig. 9.23).

Because the first clinically detectable lesion is often seen at the CEJ, the disease has also been described as feline neck lesions, cervical line lesions, or feline caries. However, ORL should not be confused with dental caries. Early caries is a passive inorganic demineralisation of the enamel, while odontoclastic resorption occurs as

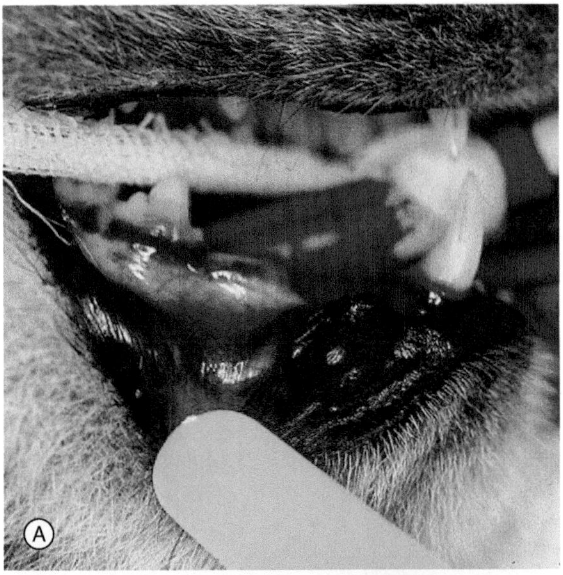

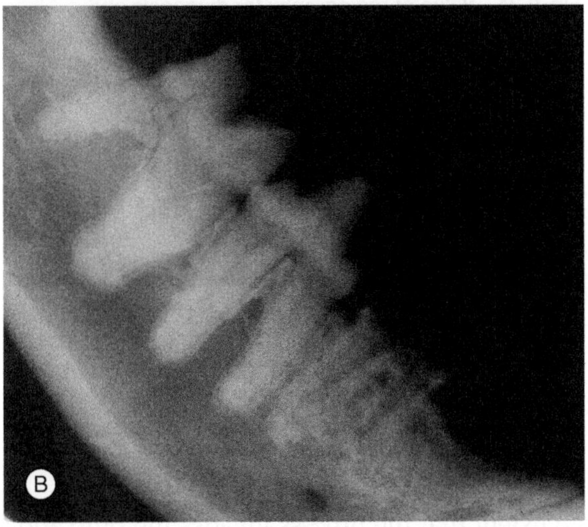

Fig. 9.22 Missing tooth with gingival overgrowth.
A: Clinical appearance. The right mandibular 3rd premolar is absent on clinical examination. The overlying gingiva is not inflamed.
B: Radiographic appearance. The roots are retained in the alveolar bone. The roots are showing evidence of ongoing resorption. The only treatment required is clinical and radiographic monitoring, i.e. there is no indication to extract the retained roots.

an active progressive destruction of the dental tissues by clastic cells. Moreover, dental caries has never been described in the cat.

All types of teeth in the feline dentition may be affected by ORLs, but lesions seem more

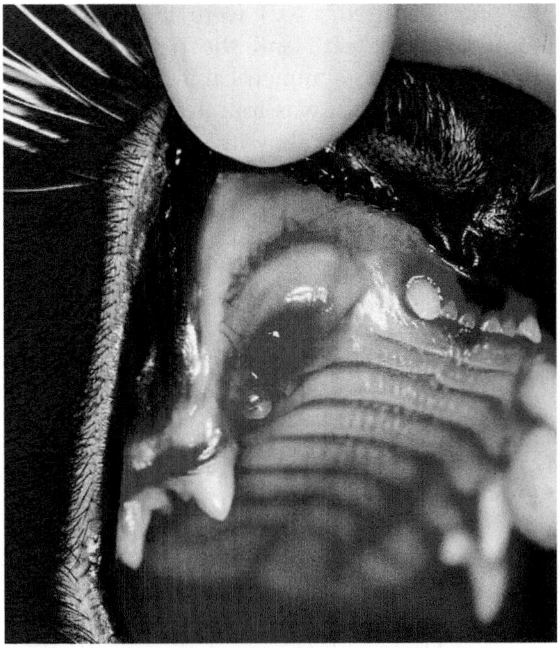

Fig. 9.23 Missing tooth with gingival inflammation. In this patient, the progressive dentine destruction has weakened and undermined the crown of the right maxillary canine tooth to such an extent that minor trauma, e.g. during chewing, has caused it to fracture, leaving the root in the alveolar bone. The gingiva overlying the retained root remnant is inflamed. The retained root remnant needs to be extracted.

common in certain teeth (Van Wessum et al, 1992; Ingham et al, 2001). The manifest lesions can often be diagnosed clinically by visual and tactile examination. As already mentioned, they commonly present as a cavity at the CEJ of the tooth. Studies, which included radiography (Ingham et al, 2001; Lindskog & Hammarström, 1980; Verstraete et al, 1998), have demonstrated that the resorption can occur anywhere on the root surfaces, i.e. not only at the CEJ. Clinical methods will only detect lesions that involve the crown, while radiography will also detect lesions confined to the root. Thus, the prevalence of ORL in studies that include radiography is higher.

In a recent study (Ingham et al, 2001), which investigated the incidence of ORL in a clinically healthy population of 228 cats (mean age was 4.92 years), using a combination of clinical examination and radiography, it was found that the overall prevalence rate was 29%. The mandibular

3rd premolars (307, 407) were the most commonly affected teeth and the pattern of ORL development was symmetrical in most cats. The risk of having ORL was found to increase with increasing age and cats with clinically missing teeth were more likely to have ORL. Neutering, sex, age at neutering or mean whole mouth gingivitis index did not affect the prevalence of ORL.

Radiography is required to identify the presence of ORL. The lesions can be detected by means of a combination of:

- Visual inspection
- Tactile examination with a dental explorer
- Radiography

Visual inspection and tactile examination with a dental explorer will only identify end-stage lesions, i.e. when the process is involving the crown and has resulted in an obvious cavity (Figs 9.20 and 9.21A). Radiography will identify lesions that are localised to the root surfaces within the alveolar bone (Fig. 9.24), which would not be detected by clinical methods. Moreover, it is only with the aid of radiography that the extent of a resorptive process can be identified (Figs 9.21B and 9.24). Selection of best treatment option thus depends on radiography. In fact, a series of full mouth radiographs (the technique is covered in Ch. 7) is recommended for all cats presented for dental therapy. If taking a series of full mouth radiographs is not possible, e.g. financial restrictions, then take one view of each mandibular premolar/molar region. The mandibular 3rd premolars are the most commonly affected teeth. If radiographs show resorption of these teeth, then a full mouth series must be taken.

The aim of any treatment is to relieve pain, prevent progression of pathology and restore function. It remains a matter of debate as to whether feline ORL cause discomfort or pain to the affected individual. Based on the fact that pulpal inflammation occurs late in the disease process, it seems likely that lesions that are limited to the root surfaces and do not communicate with the oral environment are asymptomatic. However, once dentine destruction has progressed to such an extent that the process invades the pulp and/or a communication with the oral cavity has been established (when the enamel has been resorbed or it has fractured off to reveal the dentine to the oral cavity), then discomfort and/or pain are likely. Some cats may show clinical signs indicating oral discomfort or pain, e.g. changes in food preferences (soft rather than hard diet), reduced food intake, but most cats do not.

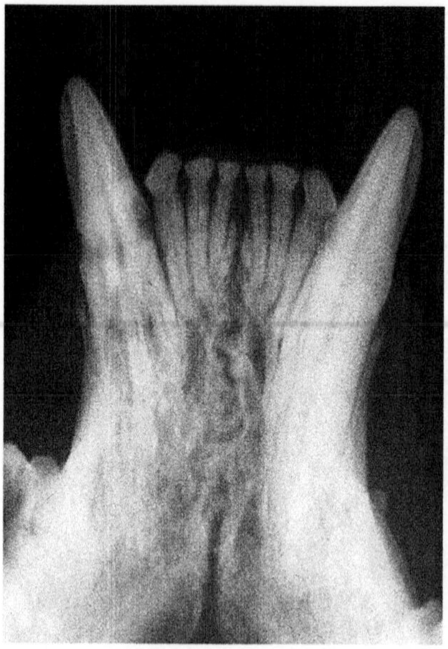

Fig. 9.24 Value of radiography for diagnosis and treatment selection. Radiography will identify lesions that are localised to the root surfaces within the alveolar bone, which would not be detected by clinical methods. Consequently, radiography is required for diagnosis of ORL. Moreover, it is only with the aid of radiography that the extent of the resorption can be evaluated.

In the radiograph depicted, the left lower canine has a resorbing root, where the process has not yet extended into the crown dentine. In fact, there was no clinical evidence of ORL. The left lower canine could thus be treated conservatively. In contrast, in the right lower canine tooth, the process has progressed to involve the crown and most of the root has been resorbed and replaced by bone-like tissue. Extraction is not possible and coronal amputation becomes the treatment of choice.

To date, there is no known treatment that prevents development and/or progression of feline ORL. It seems unlikely that such treatment can be developed without knowledge of the cause of the pathology. Currently, the suggested methods of managing odontoclastic resorptive lesions are:

- Conservative management
- Tooth extraction
- Coronal amputation

Restoration of the tooth surface has been recommended for the treatment of accessible lesions that extend into the dentine and do not involve pulp tissue. Several studies have shown that tooth resorption continues and the restorations are lost (Hopewell-Smith, 1930; Okuda & Harvey, 1992; Shigeyana et al, 1996). Consequently, the use of restoration of feline odontoclastic lesions as a major treatment technique cannot be recommended.

Conservative management consists of monitoring the lesions clinically and radiographically. This approach is recommended for lesions that are not evident on clinical examination, i.e. only seen radiographically and there is no evidence of discomfort or pain. As most lesions are only diagnosed when pathology is extensive, conservative management is rarely indicated in the general practice situation. In fact, conservative management should only be considered for canine teeth where the resorptive process is limited to the root with no oral communication.

In most cases, extraction or coronal amputation of an affected tooth is indicated. With extraction, the whole tooth is removed. This is the gold standard. However, when the root has been extensively resorbed it is often not possible to extract all tooth substance (Fig. 9.24) and coronal amputation is indicated. Preoperative radiographs are mandatory to allow selection of the appropriate treatment option.

FELINE CHRONIC GINGIVOSTOMATITIS

Feline chronic gingivostomatitis (FCGS) is a poorly defined syndrome of unknown aetiology, characterised by focal or diffuse chronic inflammation of the gingiva and oral mucosa (Gaskell & Gruffydd-Jones, 1977; Johnessee & Hurvitz, 1983; Williams & Aller, 1992). Commonly described clinical findings in cats with FCGS include elevated serum globulins, predominantly hypergammaglobulinaemia (White et al, 1992; Zetner et al, 1989) and a submucosal inflammatory infiltrate consisting of plasma cells, lymphocytes, macrophages and neutrophils (Johnessee & Hurvitz, 1983; Hennet, 1997; Reindel et al, 1987). The elevated serum globulins in affected cats and the nature of the submucosal inflammatory infiltrate have led a number of authors to suggest that there may be an immunological basis for the condition (Johnessee & Hurvitz, 1983; Williams & Aller, 1992; Sato et al, 1996). To date, no underlying intrinsic immunological abnormality in cats affected by FCGS has been identified; however, the condition may still be immune-mediated. Clinical studies have implicated the potential involvement of various viral agents, calicivirus in particular (Gruffydd-Jones, 1991; Knowles et al, 1989, 1991; Tenorio et al, 1991; Thompson et al, 1984; Waters et al, 1993; Yamamoto et al, 1989) as well as Gram-negative anaerobic bacterial species (Love et al, 1989; Sims et al, 1990). However, attempts to reproduce the disease using these putative infective aetiological agents have been unsuccessful.

FCGS can present clinically as focal or diffuse inflammation. Patterns of clinical presentation have been identified as follows (Harvey, 1990):

1. *Gingivitis with stomatitis* (Fig. 9.25). The gingival inflammation extends past the mucogingival junction onto the buccal and less often palatal/lingual mucosa. Lesions are usually symmetrical and the premolar and molar regions are likely to be more inflamed than the incisor and canine regions.
2. *Stomatitis with gingivitis* (Fig. 9.26). The inflammatory reaction is more intense in the rest of the oral mucous membranes than in the actual gingivae. In particular, the palatoglossal folds are inflamed, but there may be extensive ulceration or granulation of the gingival and/or buccal mucosa. The mucosa of the hard palate or the tongue is rarely affected. Affected cats are more likely to exhibit signs of oral discomfort than cats with predominantly gingivitis.

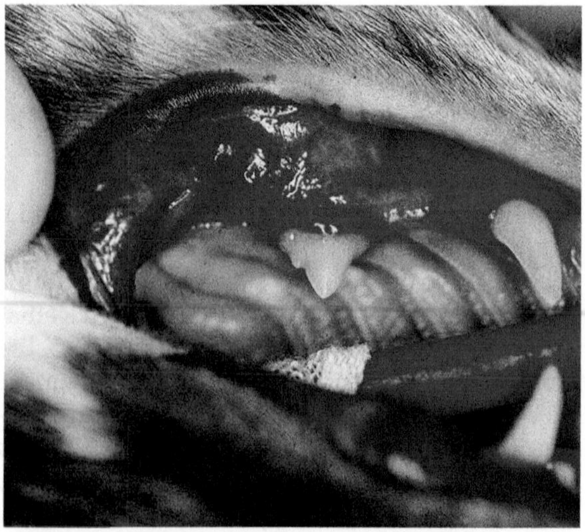

Fig. 9.25 Gingivitis with stomatitis. The gingival inflammation extends past the mucogingival junction onto the buccal and less often palatal/lingual mucosa.

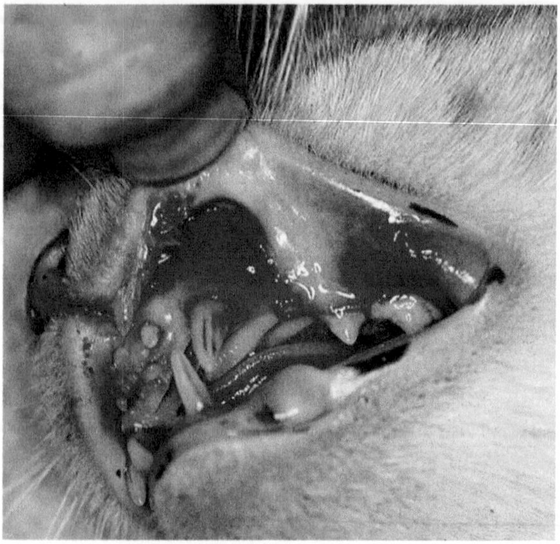

Fig. 9.26 Stomatitis with gingivitis. The inflammatory reaction is more intense in the rest of the oral mucous membranes than in the actual gingivae. Affected cats are more likely to exhibit signs of oral discomfort than are cats with predominantly gingivitis.

3. *Faucitis* (Fig. 9.27). The term 'faucitis' is a misnomer. By definition the 'fauces' is the region *medial* to the palatoglossal folds. The inflammation, which is commonly called 'faucitis', is largely confined to the palatoglossal folds and regions *lateral* to the folds. On close inspection, there is nearly always also evidence of gingivitis in the premolar and molar regions.

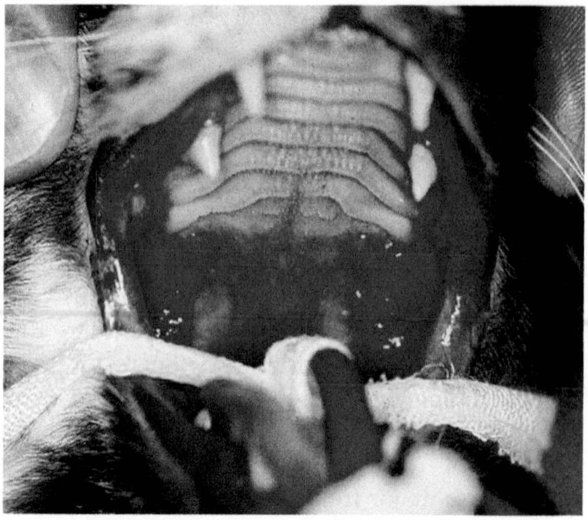

Fig. 9.27 'Faucitis'. The term 'faucitis' is a misnomer. By definition the 'fauces' is the region *medial* to the palatoglossal folds. The inflammation that is commonly called 'faucitis' is largely confined to the palatoglossal folds and regions *lateral* to the folds. On close inspection, there is nearly always also evidence of gingivitis in the premolar and molar regions.

Note that these are patterns of distribution rather than distinct diagnoses. There is often overlap with a patient presenting with one or all of these patterns.

Cats with chronic stomatitis require a thorough work-up prior to any treatment. The purpose of the work-up is not to reach a diagnosis per se, but rather an attempt to identify possible underlying causes. Such a work-up includes testing for feline immunodeficiency virus (FIV) and feline leukaemia virus (FeLV), routine haematology and blood biochemistry and sometimes biopsy and microscopic examination of the affected tissues. Radiographic evaluation to identify the presence of odontoclastic resorptive lesions, retained root remnants or other lesions is mandatory. Systemic diseases, e.g. chronic renal failure and diabetes mellitus, which may predispose to the development of severe gingival inflammation in the presence of plaque, must also be excluded before any treatment is initiated.

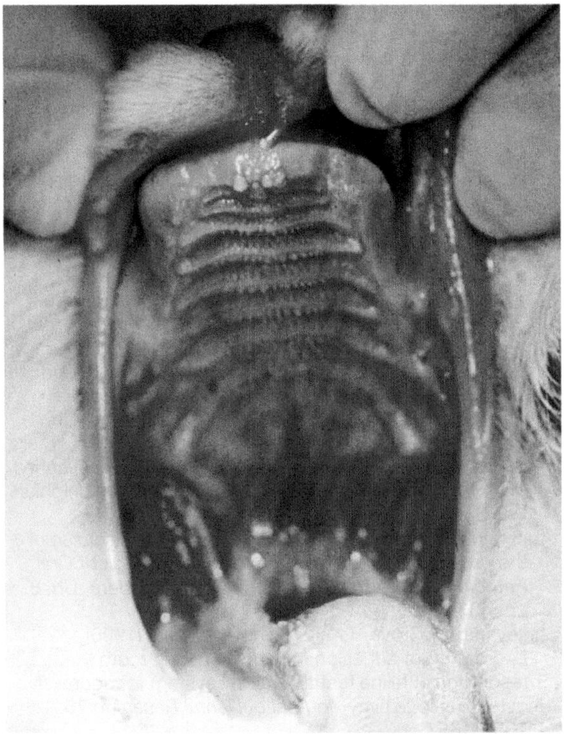

Fig. 9.28 Outcome of a radical extraction procedure. One month after radical extraction (all teeth except two upper incisors), the mucous membranes of the oral cavity are no longer inflamed. The two incisors were retained at the request of the owner who felt uncomfortable about her cat losing all its teeth. This cat still eats a hard diet, but does require assistance with grooming.

Historically, the intractable nature of the disease, in combination with a poor understanding of the aetiopathogenesis of FCGS, has resulted in the widespread use of empirical symptomatic treatment regimens; however, their efficiency has rarely been documented. In a recent study, various treatment regimens, including chlorhexidine rinses, antibiotics, corticosteroids and gold salts, were investigated over a six-month period (Harley et al, 1999). In the short term, methylprednisolone was shown to be the most effective regimen. Over the long period, the individual clinical responses were found to be diverse and none of the treatment regimens demonstrated superiority. Interferon is currently being advocated as treatment for FCGS. The data to support its efficacy are not available as yet. Interferon should not be used without a full diagnostic work-up, including viral testing. Moreover, it should not be used in the absence of remedial dental therapy, e.g. extraction of diseased teeth.

Thirty cats with FCGS were treated by extraction of most or all of the premolar and molar teeth (Hennet, 1997). Twenty-four of the 30 cats (80%) were significantly improved or clinically cured at the time of follow-up, 11–24 months following treatment.

Based on the above studies, the current treatment recommendations for cats with FCGS include a combination of periodontal therapy and a home care regimen whereby plaque accumulation is kept to a minimum. In some cats, this may result in a reduction in inflammation. Unfortunately, many cats will not cooperate adequately with home care measures and plaque reforms beyond a critical level. These cats need extraction of premolar and molar teeth. In some cats, all teeth may require removal (Fig. 9.28).

Summary

- It is useful to have a good knowledge of common oral conditions so that you can mark them adequately on the dental chart
- A variety of developmental disorders occur commonly, including missing teeth, supernumerary teeth, fused teeth, aberrant root shapes and numbers and enamel hypoplasia
- Caries (dental decay) is a recognised entity in dogs but not in cats
- Pulp and periapical conditions always require treatment by extraction or endodontic therapy

REFERENCES

Aitchison, J. (1963) Changing incisor dentition of bull dogs. *Veterinary Record* **75**: 153.

Andrews, A.H. (1972) A case of partial anodontia in a dog. *Veterinary Record* **90**: 144–145.

Arnall, L. (1960) Some aspects of dental development in the dog – II Eruption and extrusion. *Journal of Small Animal Practice* **1**: 259.

Arnbjerg, J. (1996) Idiopathic dental root replacement resorption in old dogs. *Journal of Veterinary Dentistry* **13**(3): 97–99.

Berger, M., Schawalder, P., Stich, H. et al (1996) Feline dental resorptive lesions in captive and wild leopards and lions. *Journal of Veterinary Dentistry* **13**(1): 13–21.

Clarke, D.E. & Cameron, A. (1997) Feline dental resorptive lesions in domestic and feral cats and the possible link with diet. In: *Proceedings of the 5th World Veterinary Dental Congress*, Birmingham, UK, pp. 33–34.

Crossley, D., Dubielzig, R. & Benson, K. (1997) Caries and odontoclastic resorptive lesions in a chinchilla *(Chinchilla lanigera)*. *Veterinary Record* **141**: 337–339.

Gaskell, R.M. & Gruffydd-Jones, T.J. (1977) Intractable feline stomatitis. *Veterinary Annual* **17**: 195–199.

Gorrel, C. (2003) Fluoride's role in veterinary dentistry. *Veterinary Times* **33**(43): 4–5.

Gorrel, C. & Robinson, J. (1995) Periodontal therapy and extraction technique. In: Crossley, D.A. & Penman, S. (eds) *Manual of Small Animal Dentistry*. Cheltenham: BSAVA, Ch. 14, pp. 139–149.

Gruffydd-Jones, T.J. (1991) Gingivitis and stomatitis. In: August, J.R. (ed) *Consultations in Feline Internal Medicine*. Philadelphia: WB Saunders, pp. 387–402.

Gunnraj, M.N. (1999) Dental root resorption. *Oral Surgery* **88**: 47–53.

Harley, R., Gruffydd-Jones, T.J. & Day, M.J. (1999) Clinical and immunological findings in feline chronic gingivostomatitis. In: *Proceedings of the 11th British Veterinary Dental Associations's Annual Scientific Meeting*, Birmingham, UK.

Harvey, C.E. (1990) Feline oral pathology, diagnosis and management, In: Crossley, D.A. & Penman, S. (eds) *Manual of Veterinary Dentistry*. Cheltenham: BSAVA, Ch. 13, pp. 129–138.

Harvey, C.E. & Emily, P. (1993) Occlusion, occlusive abnormalities, and orthodontic treatment. In: *Small Animal Dentistry*. St Louis, MO: Mosby, Ch. 8, pp. 266–296.

Hennet, P.R. (1997) Chronic gingivo-stomatitis in cats: Long term follow-up of 30 cases treated by dental extractions. *Journal of Veterinary Dentistry* **14**(1): 15–21.

Hopewell-Smith, A. (1930) The process of osteolysis and odontolysis, or so-called 'absorption' of calcified tissues: a new and original investigation. The evidences in the cat. *Dental Cosmos* **72**: 1036–1048.

Ingham, K.E., Gorrel, C., Blackburn, J.M. et al (2001) Prevalence of odontoclastic resorptive lesions in a clinically healthy cat population. *Journal of Small Animal Practice* **42**: 439–443.

Johnessee, J.S. & Hurvitz, A.I. (1983) Feline plasma cell gingivitis-pharyngitis. *Journal of the American Animal Hospital Association* **19**: 179–181.

Knowles, J.O., Gaskell, R.M., Gaskell, C.J. et al (1989) Prevalence of feline calicivirus, feline leukaemia virus and antibodies to FIV in cats with chronic stomatitis. *Veterinary Record* **124**: 336–338.

Knowles, J.O., McArdle, F., Dawson, S. et al (1991) Studies on the role of feline calicivirus in chronic stomatitis in cats. *Veterinary Microbiology* **27**: 205–219.

Levin, J. (1996) Tooth resorption in a Siberian tiger. In: *Proceedings of the 10th Annual Veterinary Dental Forum*, Houston, Texas, pp. 212–214.

Lindskog, S. & Hammarström, L. (1980) Evidence in favour of an anti-invasion factor in cementum or periodontal membrane. *Scandinavian Journal of Dental Research* **88**: 161–163.

Love, D.N., Johnson, J.L. & Moore, L.V. (1989) Bacteroides species from the oral cavity and oral associated diseases of cats. *Veterinary Microbiology* **19**(3): 275–281.

Okuda, A. & Harvey, C.E. (1992) Etiopathogenesis of feline dental resorptive lesions. In: Harvey, C.E. (ed) *Feline Dentistry. Veterinary Clinics of North America: Small Animal Practice*. Philadelphia: WB Saunders, pp. 1385–1404.

Reindel, J.F., Trapp, A.L., Armstrong, P.J. et al (1987) Recurrent plasmacytic stomatitis-pharyngitis in a cat with esophagitis, fibrosing gastritis and gastric nematodiasis. *Journal of the American Veterinary Medical Association* **190**(1): 65–67.

Sato, R., Inanami, O., Tanaka, Y. et al (1996) Oral administration of bovine lactoferrin for treatment of intractable stomatitis in feline immunodeficiency virus (FIV)-positive and FIV-negative cats. *American Journal of Veterinary Research* **57**(10): 1443–1446.

Shafer, W.G., Hine, M.K. & Levy, B.M. (1974a) Cysts and tumors of odontogenic origin. In: *A Textbook of Oral Pathology*, 3rd edn. Philadelphia: WB Saunders, Ch. 4, pp. 236–284.

Shafer, W.G., Hine, M.K. & Levy, B.M. (1974b) Dental caries. In: *A Textbook of Oral Pathology*, 3rd edn. Philadelphia: WB Saunders, Ch. 7, pp. 366–432.

Shafer, W.G., Hine, M.K. & Levy, B.M. (1974c) Diseases of the pulp and periapical tissues. In: *A Textbook of Oral Pathology*, 3rd edn. Philadelphia: WB Saunders, Ch. 8, pp. 433–462.

Shigeyana, Y., Grove, T.K., Strayhorn, C. et al (1996) Expression of adhesion molecules during tooth resorption in feline teeth: A model system for aggressive osteoclastic activity. *Journal of Dental Research* **75**: 1650–1657.

Sims, T.J., Moncla, B.J. & Page, R.C. (1990) Serum antibody response to antigens of oral gram-negative bacteria in cats with plasma cell gingivitis-stomatitis. *Journal of Dental Research* **69**(3): 877–882.

Skrentary, T.T. (1964) Preliminary study of the inheritance of missing teeth in the dog. *Wiener Tierarztliche Monatsschrift* **51**: 231.

Stafne, E.C. & Gibilisco, J.A. (1975a) Cysts of the jaws. In: *Oral Roentgenographic Diagnosis*, 4th edn. Philadelphia: WB Saunders, pp. 147–168.

Stafne, E.C. & Gibilisco, J.A. (1975b) Malposition of teeth. In: *Oral Roentgenographic Diagnosis*, 4th edn. Philadelphia: WB Saunders, Ch. 13, pp. 44–56.

Stafne, E.C., & Gibilisco, J.A. (1975c) The pulp cavity. In: *Oral Roentgenographic Diagnosis*, 4th edn. Philadelphia: WB Saunders, Ch. 5, pp. 61–70.

Stafne, E.C. & Gibilisco, J.A. (1975d) Dental caries. In: *Oral Roentgenographic Diagnosis*, 4th edn. Philadelphia: WB Saunders, Ch. 6, pp. 71–73.

Tenorio, A.T., Franti, C.E., Madewell, B.R. et al (1991) Chronic oral infection of cats and their relationship to persistent oral carriage of feline calici, immunodeficiency, or leukaemia viruses. *Veterinary Immunology and Immunopathology* **29**(1–2): 1–14.

Thompson, R.R., Wilcox, G.E., Clark, W.T. & Jansen, K.L. (1984) Association of calicivirus infection with chronic gingivitis and pharyngitis in cats. *Journal of Small Animal Practice* **25**: 207–210.

Van Wessum, R., Harvey, C.E. & Hennet, P. (1992) Feline dental resorptive lesions. Prevalence patterns. In: Harvey, C.E. (ed) *Feline Dentistry. Veterinary Clinics of North America: Small Animal Practice*. Philadelphia: WB Saunders, pp. 1405–1416.

Verstraete, F. (1995) Advanced oral surgery in small carnivores. In: Crossley, D.A. & Penman, S. (eds) *Manual of Small Animal Dentistry*. Cheltenham: BSAVA, Ch. 18, pp. 193–207.

Verstraete, F.J.M., Ligthelm, A.J. & Weber, A. (1992) The histological nature of epulides in dogs. *Journal of Comparative Pathology* **106**: 169–182.

Verstraete, F.J.M., Aarde Van, R.J., Nieuwoudt, B.A. et al (1996) The dental pathology of feral cats on Marion Island, Part II: periodontitis, external odontoclastic resorptive lesions and mandibular thickening. *Journal of Comparative Pathology* **115**: 283–297.

Verstraete, F.J.M., Kass, P.H. & Terpak, C.H. (1998) Diagnostic value of full mouth radiography in cats. *American Journal of Veterinary Research* **59**: 692–695.

Waters, L., Hoper, C.D., Gruffydd-Jones, T.J. et al (1993) Chronic gingivitis in a colony of cats infected with feline immunodeficiency virus and feline calicivirus. *Veterinary Record* **132**(14): 340–342.

White, S.D., Rosychuk, R.A., Reinke, S.I. et al (1992) Plasma cell stomatitis-pharyngitis in cats: 40 cases (1973–1991). *Journal of the American Veterinary Medical Association* **200**(9): 1377–1380.

Williams, C.A. & Aller, M.S. (1992) Gingivitis/stomatitis in cats. In: Harvey, C.E. (ed) *Feline Dentistry. Veterinary Clinics of North America: Small Animal Practice*. Philadelphia: WB Saunders, pp. 1361–1383.

Yamamoto, J.K., Hansen, H., Ho, E.W. et al (1989) Epidemiologic and clinical aspects of feline immunodeficiency virus infection in cats from the continental United States and Canada and possible mode of transmission. *Journal of the American Veterinary Medical Association* **194**(2): 213–220.

Zetner, K., Kampfer, P., Lutz, H. & Harvey, C. (1989) Comparative immunological and virological studies of chronic oral diseases in cats. *Wiener Tierarztliche Monatsschrift* **76**: 303–308.

10

Preventive dentistry

Oral and dental conditions generally cause distress; many cause debilitating pain to the affected animal. Most owners do not routinely examine their pet's mouth and diseases are generally not diagnosed until late in the disease process, when the animal is showing obvious signs of oral discomfort or pain.

Prevention is always preferable to treatment and many oral and dental conditions are readily amenable to preventive measures. Common conditions that can be prevented (totally or partially) include:

- Periodontal disease
- Caries
- Excessive wear
- Tooth fracture
- Certain types of malocclusion

PERIODONTAL DISEASE

The epidemiology, aetiology, pathogenesis and treatment of periodontal disease are detailed in Chapter 8. This chapter will deal with preventive measures that should be encouraged for every dog and cat.

Prevention (and treatment) of periodontal disease has two components:

- Maintenance of oral hygiene
- Professional periodontal therapy

Maintenance of oral hygiene is performed by the pet owner in the home of the animal. It is also called 'home care'. The goal of home care is to remove or, at least, reduce the accumulation of dental plaque on the tooth surfaces, i.e. plaque control. The prevention and long-term control of periodontal disease requires adequate plaque control by means of home care strategies.

Professional periodontal therapy (detailed in Ch. 8) is performed under general anaesthesia and includes:

- Supra- and subgingival scaling
- Root planing
- Tooth polishing
- Subgingival lavage
- Extraction of unsalvageable teeth
- Periodontal surgery in specific situations

The benefit of any professional periodontal therapy is short-lived unless maintained by effective home care. In fact, if no home care is instituted after professional periodontal therapy, then plaque will rapidly reform and disease will progress. It has been shown that by three months after periodontal therapy, gingivitis scores are equivalent to those recorded prior to therapy, if no home care is instituted (Gorrel & Bierer, 1999).

Maintenance of oral hygiene

Client education

The cause (dental plaque) and effects (discomfort, pain, chronic focus of infection, loss of teeth, possibility of systemic complications) of periodontal disease must be thoroughly explained to the pet owner. The owner must be made aware that home care is the most essential component in both preventing and treating periodontal disease. The responsibility of maintaining oral hygiene, i.e. keeping plaque accumulation to a level compatible with periodontal health, rests with the owner of the pet. Once instituted, home care regimens need continuous monitoring and reinforcement. The veterinary nurse and technician can play a vital role in educating clients, checking compliance and reinforcing the need for home care.

However, the owner must realise that even with home care, most animals will still need to have their teeth cleaned professionally at intervals. The intervals between professional cleaning need to be determined for each animal. With good home care, the interval between professional cleanings can be greatly extended. It is useful to draw an analogy to the situation in humans, i.e. most of us do brush our teeth daily but still require dental examinations and professional periodontal therapy (at a minimum, scaling and polishing) at regular intervals.

Toothbrushing

Toothbrushing is known to be the single most effective means of removing plaque. Studies have shown that in dogs with experimentally induced gingivitis (Tromp et al, 1986) or naturally occurring gingivitis (Gorrel & Rawlings, 1996a), daily toothbrushing

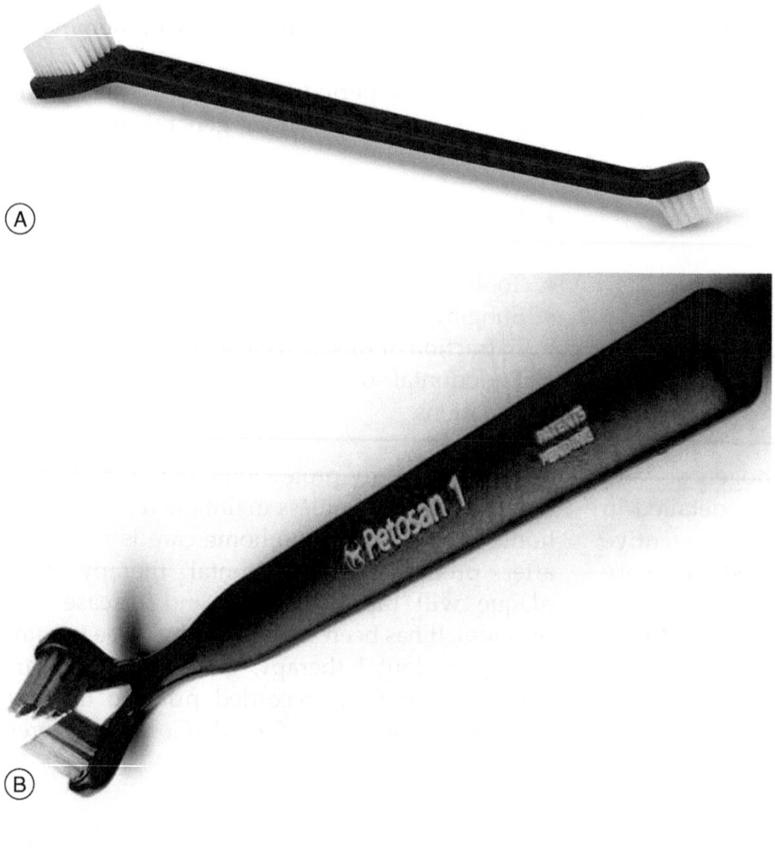

Fig. 10.1 Veterinary toothbrushes.
A: This soft nylon bristle brush has a large and a small head. The small head is useful for small dogs and cats, but also for areas that are difficult to access even in larger dogs, e.g. buccal surface of the maxillary 2nd molar.
B: The double-headed toothbrush depicted cleans the buccal as well as the palatal/lingual surfaces at the same time. It is available in three sizes, according to the size of the pet. (Slide courtesy of Petosan.)

is effective in returning the gingivae to health. In a four-year study using the beagle dog (Lindhe et al, 1975) it was shown that with no oral hygiene, plaque accumulated rapidly along the gingival margin with gingivitis developing within a few weeks. Dogs that were fed an identical diet under identical conditions but were subjected to daily toothbrushing developed no clinical signs of gingivitis. In the group that were not receiving daily toothbrushing, gingivitis progressed to periodontitis in most individuals.

Toothbrushing is the gold standard for plaque control. Every effort should be made to get every pet owner to commit to brushing their pet's teeth on a daily basis. The success of toothbrushing depends on pet cooperation and owner motivation and technical ability. Toothbrushing should be introduced gradually and as early in the animal's life as possible. Adult cats are generally less amenable to the introduction of toothbrushing than adult dogs, but with patience and persistence, many will accept some degree of home care. In contrast, kittens often accept toothbrushing more readily than puppies.

Toothbrushes. A human or veterinary toothbrush can be used. There are several brush-head and handle designs and sizes of veterinary toothbrushes available (Fig. 10.1A and B). The choice of brush should be based on the effectiveness of plaque control in the hands of each individual. In general, a soft to medium texture nylon filament brush of a suitable size for the intended pet seems to be the most comfortable.

The effectiveness of plaque removal can be assessed by applying a plaque-disclosing solution after brushing (Fig. 10.2A and B) and checking the amount of plaque still remaining on the tooth surfaces.

A flannel cloth folded over a finger, or a rubber 'finger brush' may be more comfortable for animals and owners, but is less effective (removes less plaque) than a nylon filament brush. The use of a finger brush or cloth during the training phase is useful, but every attempt should be made to get the animal to accept a proper toothbrush. There are no contraindications to careful use of an electric toothbrush, if the pet will tolerate it. In our experience, most dogs, and all cats, do not appreciate an electric toothbrush.

Toothpaste. The use of non-foaming tasty pet toothpaste is recommended, but not critical. It is the mechanical action of brushing that removes the plaque. Therefore, brushing with a toothbrush moistened with water will still do the job. However, the use of pet toothpaste is recommended as

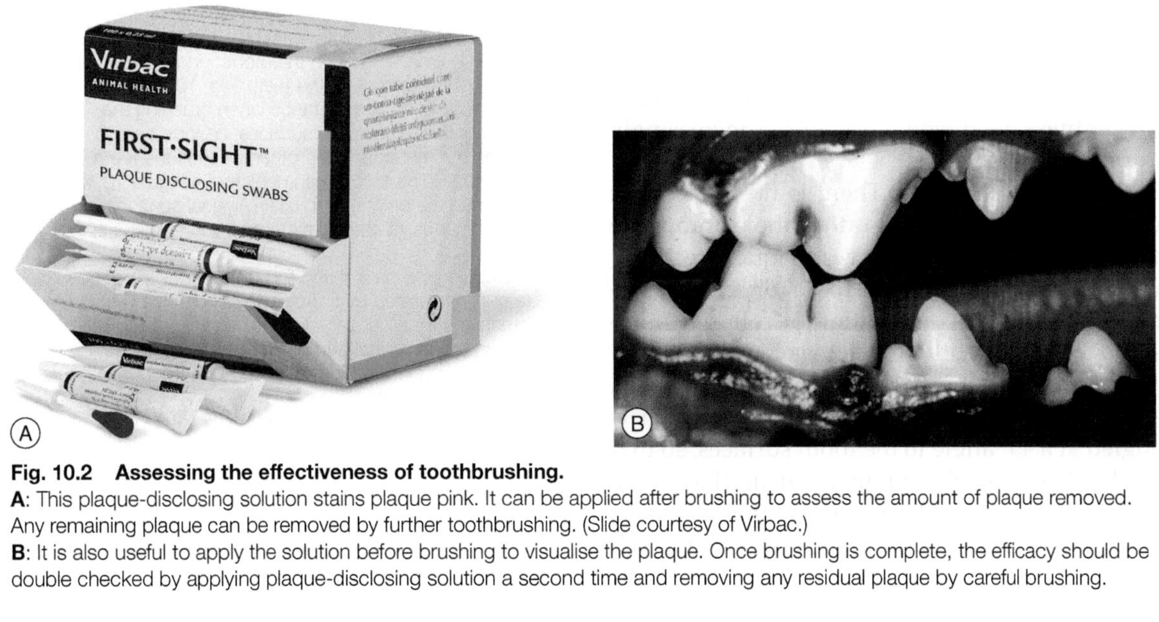

Fig. 10.2 Assessing the effectiveness of toothbrushing.
A: This plaque-disclosing solution stains plaque pink. It can be applied after brushing to assess the amount of plaque removed. Any remaining plaque can be removed by further toothbrushing. (Slide courtesy of Virbac.)
B: It is also useful to apply the solution before brushing to visualise the plaque. Once brushing is complete, the efficacy should be double checked by applying plaque-disclosing solution a second time and removing any residual plaque by careful brushing.

it tastes nice and the pet will therefore usually allow the owner to brush for longer, thus removing more plaque.

The use of a human toothpaste is not recommended, mainly due to the high fluoride content, which may lead to acute, but more likely chronic toxicity problems as our pets do not rinse and spit but will swallow the toothpaste (Gorrel, 2003).

Frequency of toothbrushing. In a study of experimental gingivitis in laboratory dogs, brushing once daily was effective in returning the gingivae to health, while brushing three times or once a week was not effective (Tromp et al, 1986). Another study has shown that brushing every other day was not sufficient to maintain clinically healthy gingivae in dogs (Gorrel & Rawlings, 1996a). Brushing twice daily with a hard human nylon filament brush resulted in traumatic gingival lesions in the dog (Sangnes, 1976).

In the only published toothbrushing study involving cats, teeth brushed either daily or twice daily on one side of the mouth had 95% less calculus, and teeth brushed once weekly had 76% less calculus than unbrushed teeth at the end of an 18-week trial period (Richardson, 1965). Unfortunately, gingivitis was not scored in this study.

Based on the above studies, the current clinical recommendation should be daily toothbrushing to establish and maintain clinically healthy gingivae for the whole life of the animal. With the increasing life expectancy of our dogs and cats, preventive medicine becomes increasingly important.

Brushing technique. There is no one correct method of brushing but rather the appropriate one that in each case removes plaque effectively without damaging either tooth or gingiva. In most instances, a combination of roll and miniscrub technique will achieve the objective.

The teeth and gingival margin are brushed in a circular or side-to-side motion. The brush is angled at a 45° angle to the tooth surfaces, so that the bristles enter the gingival sulcus (Fig. 10.3). The circling motion should ensure that all cracks and crevices in and around the teeth are cleaned.

Some practical suggestions to give to owners

- Include toothbrushing as part of the daily grooming routine. Home care is more likely to be acceptable to an older pet if it is introduced as an extension of a pre-existing routine, e.g. evening meal, walk, grooming. The owner is also more likely to remember a consistent routine
- Owners can sit small dogs and cats on their lap whilst brushing, at the same time cuddling them to reduce their apprehension; alternatively, one person cuddles and restrains whilst a second performs the toothbrushing. Some animals may better accept the use of a 'grooming table' type situation
- Start toothbrushing as early in life as possible as prevention of disease development is the goal. The primary teeth will be exfoliated and replaced by the permanent dentition. Consequently, the benefit of introducing toothbrushing at a young age will not benefit the primary teeth, but the procedure will be accepted at the time the permanent teeth erupt. Moreover, it is easier to train puppies and kittens to accept dental toothbrushing than middle-aged or older animals
- Make the animal comfortable and approach from the side rather than in front (Fig. 10.4)
- Start with just a few teeth – premolars and molars, rather than incisors, since retracting the lips is usually readily accepted, while many animals do not like having their nose lifted (Fig. 10.5). In fact, try to access the incisors without manipulating the nose excessively (Fig. 10.6)
- Gradually increase the number of teeth cleaned each time until the whole mouth can be cleaned in a single session
- Initially, the mouth does not need to be opened. Concentrate on brushing the buccal surfaces of the teeth, especially at the gingival margin
- When the animal is comfortable with having the buccal surfaces of all its teeth brushed, an attempt should be made to open the mouth and brush the palatal and lingual surfaces of the teeth (Fig. 10.7). It is useful to have assistance when brushing the palatal and lingual tooth surfaces, i.e. one person opens the mouth and the other brushes the teeth (Fig. 10.8). The toothbrush depicted in Figure 10.1B will clean the buccal and palatal/lingual surfaces simultaneously if the animal allows you to place it correctly
- If brushing the palatal and lingual surfaces is not possible (e.g. not tolerated by the pet), then continue with daily brushing of the buccal surfaces. However, gingivitis will occur on the palatal and lingual surfaces if these are not brushed (Ingham & Gorrel, 2001) and periodontitis may occur at these sites
- Apply a plaque-disclosing solution (Fig. 10.2) and brush away any remaining plaque
- Offer a reward at the end of the procedure, e.g. a game or a walk

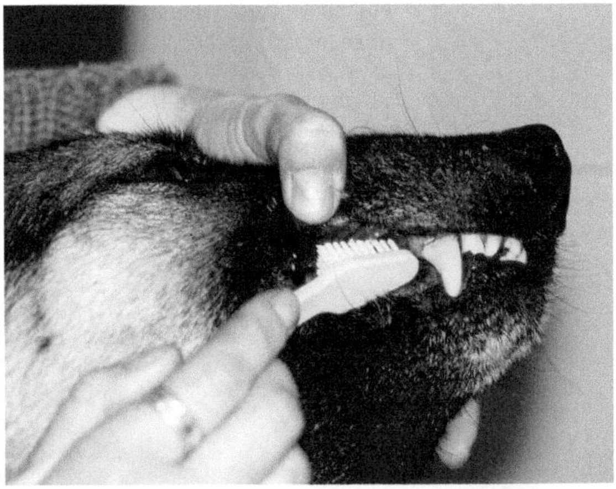

Fig. 10.3 Toothbrushing technique. Subgingival plaque is a consequence of supragingival plaque migrating in an apical direction. To remove plaque from the gingival sulcus, the toothbrush is angled at a 45° angle to the tooth surface, which allows the bristles to enter the sulcus. Even with optimal technique, toothbrushing will not clean more than 1–2 mm below the gingival margin. Consequently, the best way to prevent plaque accumulating in the sulcus is meticulous supragingival plaque control.

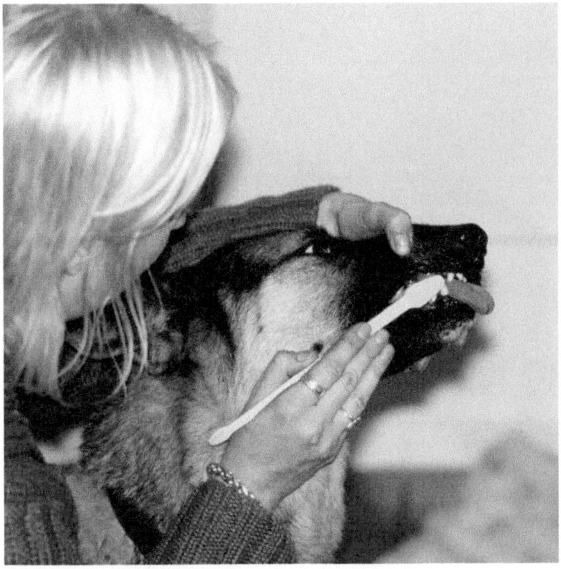

Fig. 10.4 Approach from the side rather than the front. Approaching the animal head on, armed with a toothbrush, is unlikely to be tolerated. Instead, make the pet comfortable and approach from the side.

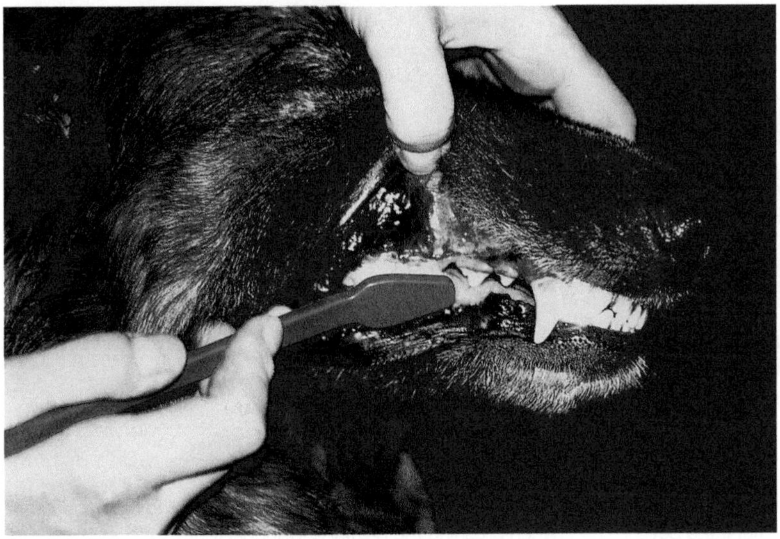

Fig. 10.5 Start with just a few teeth. Start with brushing the premolars and molars. Gradually increase the number of teeth cleaned each day until all teeth can be cleaned in one session. It usually takes two to four weeks for an animal to accept having all teeth cleaned in one sitting.

In the gingivitis and periodontitis patient, it is likely that some gingival bleeding will occur when brushing is first started. It is important to clarify to the owner that they need to carry on brushing despite the bleeding. As a result of the daily plaque removal, the gingivae will become clinically healthy and the bleeding will stop.

Dental diets and dental hygiene chews

The use of products (dental diets, hygiene chews and biscuits) aimed at encouraging chewing activity and designed with textural properties that maximise the self-cleansing effect of function are beneficial in reducing the accumulation of

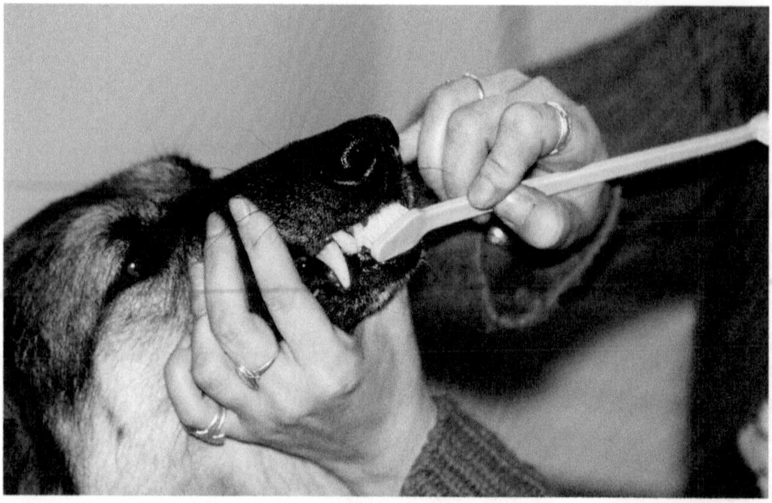

Fig. 10.6 Avoid manipulating the nose. Most dogs and cats do not like to have their nose lifted. Try to brush the incisors without manipulating the nose excessively.

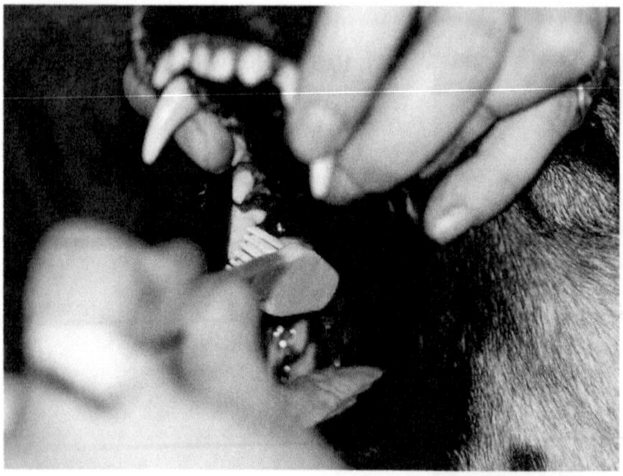

Fig. 10.7 Importance of brushing palatal and lingual tooth surfaces. Gingivitis will occur on palatal and lingual surfaces if these are not brushed. Every attempt should be made to open the mouth and access these surfaces. Many pets tolerate the double-ended toothbrush that cleans the outer and inner tooth surfaces at the same time. If the pet does not allow brushing of the palatal and lingual surfaces, carry on with daily brushing of the buccal tooth surfaces.

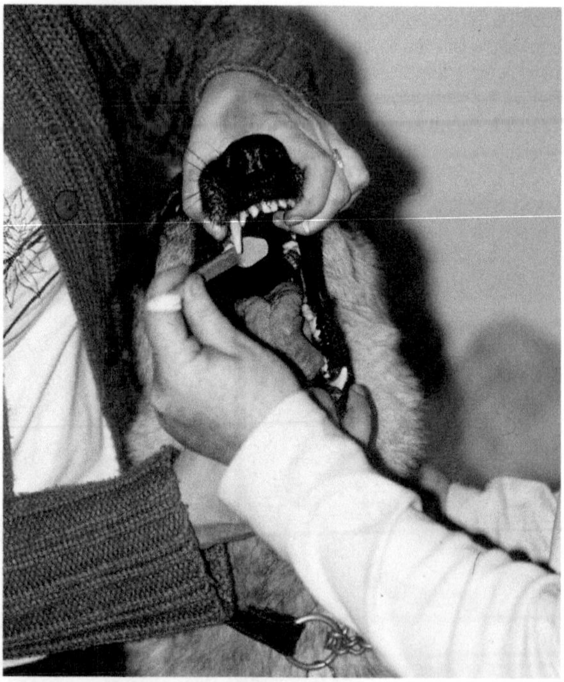

Fig. 10.8 Assistance is useful. It is useful to have assistance when brushing the palatal and lingual tooth surfaces. One person restrains the pet and opens the mouth, while the other brushes.

dental deposits and consequently the degree of gingivitis that develops.

None of the products in this category is as effective as daily toothbrushing. Consequently, their use cannot achieve or maintain clinically healthy gingivae in the absence of toothbrushing.

Periodontal disease has been linked with aspects of diet. Several studies have investigated the local effect of diet on plaque formation and development of gingivitis in the dog (Egelberg, 1965a, 1965b). A coarse diet may reduce plaque accumulation on some teeth and on some tooth surfaces. Although consumption of soft foods may promote plaque accumulation, the general belief that dry foods provide significant oral cleansing should be regarded with scepticism. In fact, one study reported that feeding a canned food performed similarly to a dry food in the degree of plaque and calculus accumulation (Boyce & Logan, 1994). In a large epidemiological survey, dogs consuming dry food did not consistently demonstrate improved periodontal health when compared with dogs eating moist foods (Harvey et al, 1996).

Specifically designed dental diets (Jensen et al, 1995; Logan et al, 2002) and dental hygiene chews (Gorrel & Rawlings, 1996b; Gorrel et al, 1998, 1999; Gorrel & Bierer, 1999; Ingham et al, 2002), with enhanced textural characteristics, have been shown to significantly reduce accumulation of dental deposits and the degree of gingivitis, in both long-term and short-term studies. It is not known whether this reduced degree of gingivitis is sufficient to prevent the development of periodontitis. Further studies of longer duration are required.

While every attempt should be made to ensure that daily toothbrushing is performed by the owner, the reduction of accumulation of dental deposits (plaque and calculus), thus reducing the severity of gingivitis by dietary means, is a useful adjunctive measure and is highly recommended to pet owners. In selecting an appropriate dental diet or dental hygiene chews, we recommend using either a product that has been shown to be effective in peer-reviewed publications, or a product that has been awarded a VOHC® Seal of Acceptance. (The Veterinary Oral Health Council (VOHC®) Seal of Acceptance system identifies products that meet pre-set standards for prevention of accumulation of dental plaque and calculus (tartar). It is a product effectiveness recognition system, with no regulatory function, and is limited to considering products designed to control plaque and calculus.)

To summarise, there is no magic bullet that we can feed our pets to prevent periodontal disease. Daily toothbrushing remains the single most effective method of restoring inflamed gingivae to health and of then maintaining clinically healthy gingivae. Compliance may be an issue for some people. Compliance failure has not been critically investigated in veterinary dentistry; however, it is not difficult to imagine that many factors may prevent owners from brushing their pets' teeth. Such factors include lack of skill, questionable perceived benefit, unpleasantness of the procedure and lifestyle (lack of time). One study evaluated compliance in a 6- to 21-month period following periodontal therapy and home care instruction (Miller & Harvey, 1994). This study reported that 53% of clients surveyed were satisfactorily compliant. However, the report was based on a telephone survey and clinical effectiveness of compliance was not assessed. Our experience is that a combination of client education, continuous reinforcement and individually determined recalls to check efficacy yields surprisingly good compliance.

CARIES

Caries occurs in the dog. It has not been described in cats.

In simple terms, caries occurs when plaque bacteria use fermentable carbohydrate (notably sugar) from the diet as a source of energy. The fermentation by-products are acidic and demineralise the enamel. Caries can thus be prevented by removing the bacteria (toothbrushing) in combination with removing their substrate (sugar and other easily fermentable carbohydrate). Dogs should not be fed human biscuits and confectionery, as they are high in sugar.

EXCESSIVE WEAR

Attrition is defined as wear of tooth surfaces that are in contact with one another and abrasion as wear of tooth surfaces that are not in contact with one another.

Excessive attrition can occur under certain circumstances. Stone chewing is a common cause of excessive attrition. Another common cause is playing with a ball on a sandy surface. The ball becomes wet and covered with sand or grit and as the animal bites on the ball, the teeth are worn excessively. Prevention in such circumstances is restricting access to stones and playing with a ball in an environment where the ball does not become covered in abrasive material.

Loss of teeth (due to disease or trauma) and malocclusion may also predispose to excessive attrition. If extensive extractions are required, the resultant occlusion must be evaluated and preventive measures instituted as appropriate.

In humans, the most common cause of abrasion is incorrect use of a toothbrush. We have not seen this type of iatrogenic injury in dogs and cats. Other causes include the ingestion of solids or liquids that are highly acidic, or the regurgitation or vomiting of acids from the stomach, which enhance the tissue destruction caused by incorrect brushing technique. In the dog, the most common cause of abrasion is cage biting. The result of the progressive loss of tooth substance is fracture (generally with pulpal exposure) of the weakened tooth. Every effort should be made to rid the animal of this habit. If this cannot be achieved, then the animal should not be caged.

TOOTH FRACTURE

The incidence of tooth fracture, especially in dogs, can be reduced by preventing certain types of behaviour by the owner and/or pet. The owner should be discouraged from behaviour such as throwing stones for the dog to collect. As already mentioned in the previous section, circumstances and/or behaviour that predispose to excessive tooth wear and weakening of the teeth should be avoided. Chewing on hard bones or toys should not be encouraged. Endodontic treatment of fractured teeth is a large proportion of the clinical case load at our referral practice and a large number of the dogs referred for treatment fractured one or several teeth by biting on hard bones or toys. Softer bones should also be avoided. These will be chewed and swallowed, often causing digestive problems, or become impacted on or between teeth. Raw bones are also potential sources of infection for animals and owners (*Sarcocystis, Campylobacter, Toxoplasma, Salmonella*).

MALOCCLUSION

Malocclusion is common and may cause pain/discomfort and severe oral pathology. Occlusal evaluation is part of the basic oral examination of a conscious animal. To make an evaluation, the practitioner needs to be able to identify normal occlusion for the species and breed and have an understanding of the aetiology and pathogenesis of malocclusion. Occlusion and malocclusion are detailed in Chapter 5. In general, the treatment of malocclusion is best left to a veterinarian with special skills in dentistry, namely expertise in endodontics and orthodontics. It is possible to prevent development of some types of malocclusion.

Preventive measures that can be performed in a general practice include:

- Extraction of persistent primary teeth
- Interceptive orthodontics
- A removable orthodontic device

General practitioners are encouraged to implement these measure.

Summary

- There is no magic bullet that we can feed our pets to prevent periodontal disease: daily toothbrushing remains the single most effective method of restoring inflamed gingivae to health and of then maintaining clinically healthy gingivae
- Compliance may be an issue for some people. Compliance failure has not been critically investigated in veterinary dentistry; however, it is not difficult to imagine that many factors may prevent owners from brushing their pets' teeth. Such factors include lack of skill, questionable perceived benefit, unpleasantness of the procedure and lifestyle (lack of time)
- One study evaluated compliance in a period of 6–21 months following periodontal therapy and home care instruction (Miller & Harvey, 1994). This study reported that 53% of clients surveyed were satisfactorily compliant. However; the report was based on a telephone survey and clinical effectiveness of compliance was not assessed
- Our experience is that a combination of client education, continuous reinforcement and individually determined recalls to check efficacy yields surprisingly good compliance
- Caries in dogs is prevented by toothbrushing and avoiding treats containing sugar
- Attrition, abrasion and tooth fracture are prevented by modifying play behaviours or the animal's environment
- Malocclusion can be prevented by extraction of persistent primary teeth, interceptive orthodontics and by the use of appropriate removable orthodontic devices
- Setting up 'dental clinics' may help with owner compliance for daily toothbrushing

REFERENCES

Boyce, E.N. & Logan, E.I. (1994) Oral health assessment in dogs: study design and results. *Journal of Veterinary Dentistry* **11**(2): 64–74.

Egelberg, J. (1965a) Local effects of diet on plaque formation and gingivitis development in dogs. III Effect of frequency of meals and tube feeding. *Odontologisk Revy* **16**: 50–60.

Egelberg, J. (1965b) Local effects of diet on plaque formation and gingivitis development in dogs. I Effect of hard and soft diets. *Odontologisk Revy* **16**: 31–41.

Gorrel, C. (2003) Fluoride's role in veterinary dentistry. *Veterinary Times* **33**(43), 10 November.

Gorrel, C. & Bierer, T. (1999) Long term effects of a dental hygiene chew on the periodontal health of dogs. *Journal of Veterinary Dentistry* **16**(3): 109–113.

Gorrel, C. & Rawlings, J.M. (1996a) The role of tooth-brushing and diet in the maintenance of periodontal health in dogs. *Journal of Veterinary Dentistry* **13**(3): 139–143.

Gorrel, C. & Rawlings, J.M. (1996b) The role of a 'dental hygiene chew' in maintaining periodontal health in dogs. *Journal of Veterinary Dentistry* **13**(1): 31–34.

Gorrel, C., Inskeep, G. & Inskeep, T. (1998) Benefits of a 'dental hygiene chew' on the periodontal health of cats. *Journal of Veterinary Dentistry* **15**(3): 135–138.

Gorrel, C., Warrick, J. & Bierer, T. (1999) Effect of a new dental hygiene chew on periodontal health in dogs. *Journal of Veterinary Dentistry* **16**(2): 77–81.

Harvey, C.E., Shofer, F.S. & Laster, L. (1996) Correlation of diet, other chewing activities and periodontal disease in North American client-owned dogs. *Journal of Veterinary Dentistry* **13**(3): 101–105.

Ingham, K.E. & Gorrel, C. (2001) Effect of long-term intermittent periodontal care on canine periodontal disease. *Journal of Small Animal Practice* **42**(2): 67–70.

Ingham, K.E., Gorrel, C. & Bierer, T.L. (2002) Effect of a dental chew on dental substrates and gingivitis in cats. *Journal of Veterinary Dentistry* **19**(4): 201–204.

Jensen, L., Logan, E.I., Finney, O. et al (1995) Reduction in accumulation of plaque, stain and calculus in dogs by dietary means. *Journal of Veterinary Dentistry* **12**(4): 161–163.

Lindhe, J., Hamp, S-E. & Löe, H. (1975) Plaque induced periodontal disease in beagle dogs. A 4-year clinical, roentgenographical and histometrical study. *Journal of Periodontal Research* **10**: 243–255.

Logan, E.I., Finney, O. & Hefferren, J. (2002) Effects of a dental food on plaque accumulation and gingival health in dogs. *Journal of Veterinary Dentistry* **19**(1): 15–18.

Miller, B.R. & Harvey, C.E. (1994) Compliance with oral hygiene recommendations following periodontal treatment in client-owned dogs. *Journal of Veterinary Dentistry* **11**(1): 18–19.

Richardson, R.L. (1965) Effect of administering antibiotics, removing the major salivary glands and toothbrushing on dental calculi formation in the cat. *Archives of Oral Biology* **10**: 245–253.

Sangnes, G. (1976) A pilot study on the effect of toothbrushing on the gingiva of a beagle dog. *Scandinavian Journal of Dental Research* **84**: 106–108.

Tromp, J.A., van Rijn, L.J. & Jansen, J. (1986) Experimental gingivitis and frequency of tooth-brushing in the beagle dog model. Clinical findings. *Journal of Clinical Periodontology* **13**: 190–194.

11

Tooth extraction

Tooth extraction is commonly indicated in small animal practice. The procedure is often time-consuming and fraught with difficulties. The risk of complications with extraction is significant. Many of the potential complications are iatrogenic and can thus be avoided.

Tooth extraction is the remit of the veterinarian. While the trained veterinary nurse and technician may legally be allowed to perform minor surgery at the request, and under the direct supervision, of the veterinarian, tooth extraction cannot be considered minor surgery (see Ch. 1). However, veterinary nurses and technicians fill a vital role in assisting the veterinarian with tooth extraction. Simple extraction usually does not require assistance, but complicated extractions generally do. The advantages of assistance include reduced trauma to the tissues and consequently better healing (in less time, with less discomfort). The role of the assisting nurse or technician includes retraction of tissues (mucoperiosteal flaps), suction, irrigation of bur (if a slow-speed unit without water cooling is being used to remove bone/section teeth), directing the light, etc. As already mentioned (Ch. 3), the person assisting in the surgical procedure should not also be the person responsible for monitoring the anaesthesia. To be able to provide the best assistance, veterinary nurses and technicians need to be familiar with the various extraction techniques available.

The purpose of this chapter is to help the veterinary nurse and technician understand the techniques used, thus enabling them to provide the best possible assistance to the veterinarian performing these procedures.

POSSIBLE COMPLICATIONS

As already mentioned, the risk of iatrogenic damage and complications is high with extractions. It is essential to know the normal anatomy of the oral cavity to prevent the surgeon from causing iatrogenic damage, e.g. severing neurovascular structures, which would result in sensory deficits and haemorrhage.

Preoperative radiographs are mandatory before extraction of a tooth. It is only with the aid of radiographs that the extent of pathology can be visualised. Also, the preoperative radiographs will allow optimal planning of extraction as the anatomy of the tooth will be visualised and most complicating factors detected. Postoperative radiographs to assess the extraction are also required.

Potential complications include:

1. *Thermal bone injury.* Adequate water-cooling of the bur (whether used in a high- or slow-speed handpiece) is mandatory. Overheating will result in damage to both soft tissue and bone. Thermal necrosis of bone usually results in the development of a bone sequestrum that needs to be surgically retrieved as a second procedure.
2. *Tooth fracture.* Extraction may result in fracture of the tooth, either the crown, or the

root. The most common cause of tooth fracture is incorrect extraction technique, e.g. using excessive force with elevators or using dental forceps without loosening the tooth sufficiently first. Every attempt should be made to extract the whole tooth. If remnants of tooth are not removed, these need to be documented radiographically and the animal rebooked for further evaluation. Moreover, the owner should always be informed and made aware that further surgery may be required.

3. *Oronasal communication.* Communication between a maxillary tooth alveolus and the nasal chamber may occur due to disease (e.g. periodontitis or periapical disease) or be iatrogenic in origin. Established fistulae are lined by epithelium and will, therefore, not heal spontaneously, but require surgical repair.

4. *Emphysema.* This can occur if the high-speed handpiece is angled so that air is blown into the bone and soft tissues. Continuous air-drying, especially if the air is directed into the alveolus, can also lead to emphysema. Cats seem particularly prone and show swelling across the base of the nose and forehead. There is obvious crepitus on palpation of the swelling. Alternatively, the floor of the mouth is swollen. The condition usually resolves itself over a few hours/days. The owners are often concerned and it is best avoided.

5. *Sublingual oedema.* Traumatising the lingual mucosa may result in sublingual oedema. If severe, it may require medical management with anti-inflammatory drugs and sometimes diuretics. It is easily avoided by using a gentle technique.

6. *Jaw fracture.* Advanced periodontitis of mandibular teeth will weaken the mandible, and jaw fractures (spontaneous and iatrogenic) can and do happen.

7. *Haemorrhage.* There is potential for extensive, potentially life-threatening haemorrhage if the major blood vessels (infraorbital artery, palatine artery, inferior alveolar artery) are transected. In addition, clotting defects are a concern and may cause life-threatening haemorrhage. Ideally, any such defects should be identified prior to surgery.

8. *Sensory deficits.* Sensory deficits will result if the nerve vessels (infraorbital, mandibular, mental) are transected during extraction. Similarly, inadvertently inserting instruments into the mandibular canal will damage the neurovascular structures, leading to postoperative pain and potentially permanent sensory deficits.

TYPES OF EXTRACTION

There are two basic extraction techniques, namely:

1. *Closed (non-surgical).* This can be defined as extraction using simple luxation and/or elevation, without the need to remove alveolar bone. Either the extraction socket is left open to heal by granulation, or it may be closed by suturing the gingiva over the defect to achieve primary healing and reduce postoperative pain.
2. *Open (surgical).* In this technique a mucoperiosteal flap is raised to access the alveolar bone. The alveolar bone overlying the buccal surface of the tooth root is usually removed to facilitate tooth removal. The mucoperiosteal flap is replaced to close the extraction socket, thus allowing primary healing.

CHOICE OF EXTRACTION TECHNIQUE

The choice of either a closed or an open technique will depend on several factors. The most important are:

1. Tooth morphology
2. Existing pathology
3. Operator preference.

Preoperative radiographs are mandatory to evaluate the tooth morphology and extent of pathology necessitating the extraction.

Situations where an open extraction technique is absolutely indicated (i.e. the tooth cannot technically be removed using a closed technique, since alveolar bone must be removed to free the root) include:

- Bizarre root morphology, with bends or spirals
- Extensive root resorption ± ankylosis
- Periodontally sound upper and lower canines (the roots are curved and wider below the cemento-enamel junction than above it)

Situations where an open technique may facilitate extraction include:

- Retained root remnants
- Any multiple-rooted tooth which is periodontally sound, i.e. there is no loss of alveolar bone (an open technique will make access to the furcation and individual roots possible)
- Feline teeth

With the exception of teeth affected by advanced periodontitis, I generally use an open extraction technique as it enables visualisation of the periodontal ligament space. Consequently, instrument placement can be more precise, the extraction is thus less traumatic to adjacent tissues and healing is more predictable. Human patients report less postoperative discomfort following an open technique than a closed technique. The same is probably true for our patients.

EXTRACTION TECHNIQUES

General considerations

Extraction of teeth is a surgical procedure. While it is not possible to achieve a sterile environment in the oral cavity, the mouth should be clean before extraction is performed. All teeth should be scaled and polished and the mouth rinsed with a chlorhexidine solution.

Good visibility simplifies the procedure greatly. A good light source is essential. In addition, the three-way syringe should be used to clean the mouth out frequently during the procedure. Suction is extremely useful and strongly recommended. Extraction is easy if the periodontal ligament space can be visualised and consequently instruments applied at the correct location. Contrary to common belief, tooth extraction does not require force. It is best achieved by planned placement of instruments and carefully working around the whole circumference of the tooth cutting the periodontal ligament, thus releasing the tooth. Equipment and instrumentation requirements for extraction are detailed in Chapter 2.

Closed extraction

Single-rooted teeth

Teeth suitable for this technique are incisors, 1st premolars and mandibular 3rd molars in the dog and maxillary 2nd premolars and 1st molars in the cat. It can also be used for canine teeth with extensive bone loss due to severe periodontitis.

Procedure

- The gingival attachment is cut around the whole circumference of the tooth using either a No. 11 or No. 15 scalpel blade in a handle or a *sharp* luxator (Figs 11.1 and 11.5A)
- A sharp luxator of appropriate size (its concave surface should equal the curvature of the root

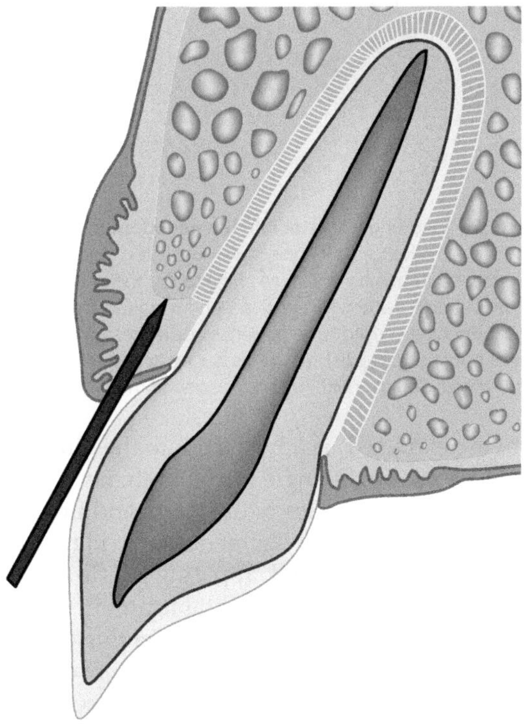

Fig. 11.1 Cutting the gingival attachment to the tooth. A scalpel blade or a sharp luxator is inserted into the gingival sulcus until the instrument contacts the margin of the alveolar bone. The gingival attachment to the tooth surface is released in this way around the whole circumference of the tooth. This is the first step of any extraction, irrespective of whether a closed or open technique is planned. There is no attempt to enter the periodontal ligament space at this stage. The purpose of this cut is just to free the gingival attachment. (Reproduced from the *Manual of Small Animal Dentistry* with kind permission from BSAVA.)

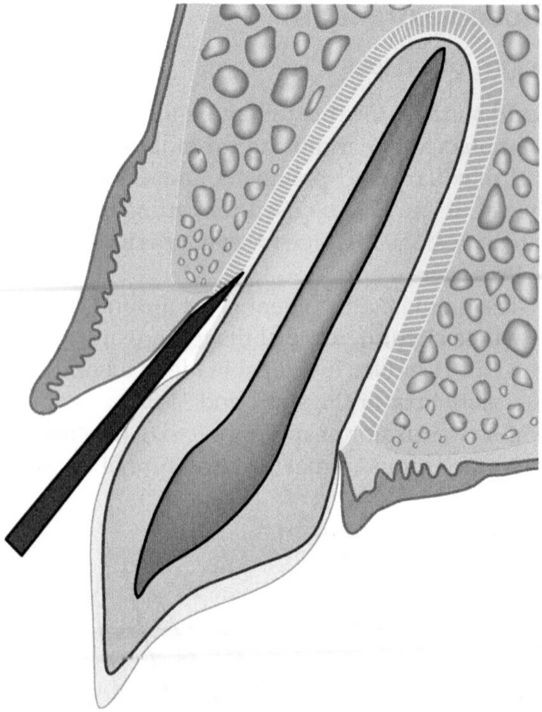

Fig. 11.2 Inserting a luxator into the periodontal ligament. The luxator is advanced into the gingival sulcus at a slight angle to the tooth, i.e. following the surface of the tooth, and pressed into the periodontal ligament space. It is worked around the whole circumference of the tooth, using gentle apical pressure, cutting the periodontal ligament fibres. (Reproduced from the *Manual of Small Animal Dentistry* with kind permission from BSAVA.)

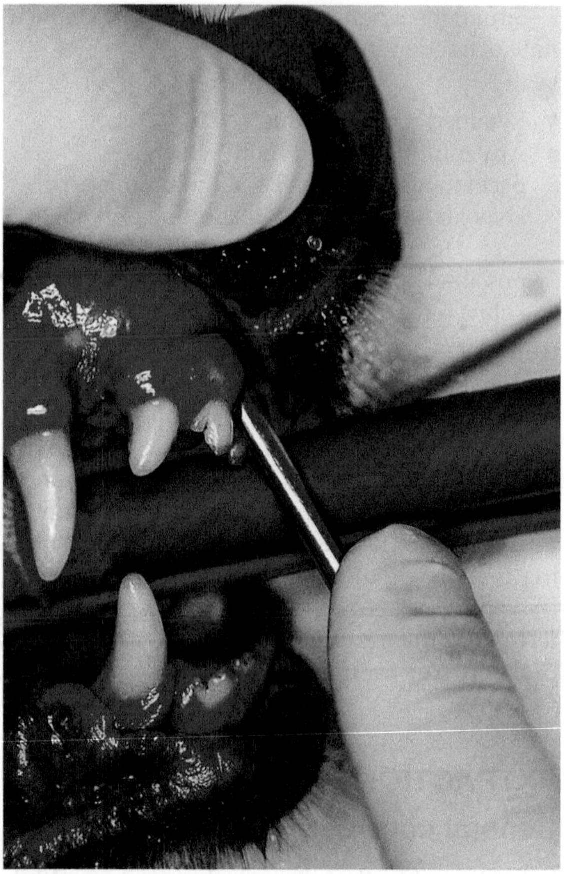

Fig. 11.3 Using a dental elevator in an apical fashion. The elevator is worked circumferentially around the tooth, with a steady gentle rotational pressure held at each point for 10–15 seconds to fatigue the deeper periodontal fibres.

being extracted) is advanced into the gingival sulcus at a slight angle to the tooth, i.e. following the surface of the tooth, and pressed into the periodontal ligament space (Fig. 11.2)

- The luxator is worked, applying gentle apical pressure, into the periodontal ligament space around the whole circumference of the tooth to cut the periodontal ligament fibres. Once sufficient space has been created between the tooth and the alveolar bone, an elevator can be used. Some veterinarians prefer to perform the whole extraction using luxators of increasing size, i.e. do not switch to elevators. This is acceptable procedure as long as the luxators are used in the correct fashion, i.e. in an apical direction, without rotation, to cut the periodontal ligament fibres. Luxators should not be rotated, as this will damage the fine end of the instrument
- The elevator is also worked circumferentially around the tooth, with a steady gentle rotational pressure held at each point for 10–15 seconds to fatigue the deeper periodontal fibres (Fig. 11.3). Haemorrhage will be created at the same time, which adds hydraulic pressure to the process of breaking down the fibres. As the periodontal ligament fibres break and the tooth begins to loosen, the elevator can be pushed further apically, and rotated more
- When the tooth is loose, it can be drawn out of the socket with fingers or forceps. In my experience, the use of dental forceps usually results in fracture of the apical portion of the root. I do not use them or recommend their use

Multiple-rooted teeth

The tooth is sectioned into single-rooted units, such that each unit can be removed as a single-rooted tooth. The reason for sectioning is that the roots of multiple-rooted teeth diverge away from each other, which gives the tooth greater stability in the mouth, but also makes it impossible to extract the tooth as a single unit.

The three-rooted teeth are the maxillary 4th premolars in the cat. In dogs, the maxillary 4th premolars, and the maxillary 1st and 2nd molars are three-rooted. All other multiple-rooted teeth have two roots. Note, however, that supernumerary roots are quite common. Preoperative radiographs will allow detection of extra roots and allow optimal sectioning into single-rooted units.

Procedure

- The gingival attachment to the tooth is cut (as described earlier)
- The furcation(s) of the roots is exposed by elevating the gingiva with a round-ended periosteal elevator
- The tooth is sectioned into single-rooted units using a bur in either a slow- or high-speed handpiece. Traditionally a 701 taper fissure cut bur has been recommended for sectioning teeth. I find fissure burs difficult to use for this purpose, unless the furcation is open (gingival recession exposing the furcation), as they do not cut efficiently when the end is used (the cutting surfaces of a fissure bur are its sides). In my hands, a better method is to use a round bur (size 4–6 for cats and 6–8 for dogs), since this can be used to cut a tunnel in the alveolar bone under the furcation before cutting up into the crown. At all times, water-cooling is essential to prevent thermal damage to surrounding tissues. An alternative to the round bur is a pear shaped bur, e.g. 331L type, which cuts both on the end and on the shank
- The single root units are luxated and elevated as already described for a single-rooted tooth. However, in addition to using the elevator in an apical direction, it can be inserted in a horizontal fashion between the tooth root and bone, and gently rotated to lift the tooth roots out of their alveoli (Fig. 11.4 A, B and C)
- Any sharp bony edges are removed with a round bur or bone cutters. The loose gingiva needs to be protected, e.g. with a plastic spatula
- Unless the gingiva lies flat against the alveolar bone after extraction, suturing the extraction socket closed should be considered to speed healing, prevent infection, and reduce postoperative pain

Open extraction

An open extraction technique can be used for all teeth.

In open extractions, a mucoperiosteal flap is raised (usually on the buccal aspect of the tooth) to expose the alveolar bone. Releasing incisions (from the gingival margin to beyond the mucogingival line) are usually placed at one or both ends of the initial incision to allow the flap to be raised past the mucogingival junction, thus exposing most of the buccal bone plate. It is essential to protect the flap during the procedure, as this is the tissue that will be used to suture over the extraction socket. Plastic spatulas or gingival retractors can be used to keep the flap intact. Having an assistant to work the spatula or retractors will make the extraction easier and quicker, as well as prevent iatrogenic damage to the flap. Once the tooth has been removed, the flap is replaced and sutured *without tension* to the palatal/lingual mucosa to close the extraction socket.

In the following, the maxillary canine tooth will be used to exemplify the details of the open extraction technique. Differences for other teeth will be highlighted as required.

Maxillary canine

Procedure

- The gingival attachment around the whole circumference of the canine is cut (Fig. 11.5A). This incision is then extended rostrally to the distal aspect of the 3rd incisor and distally to the mesial or distal aspect of the 2nd premolar using a No. 11 or No. 15 blade in a handle. This involves cutting the buccal gingival attachment of the 1st and 2nd premolars

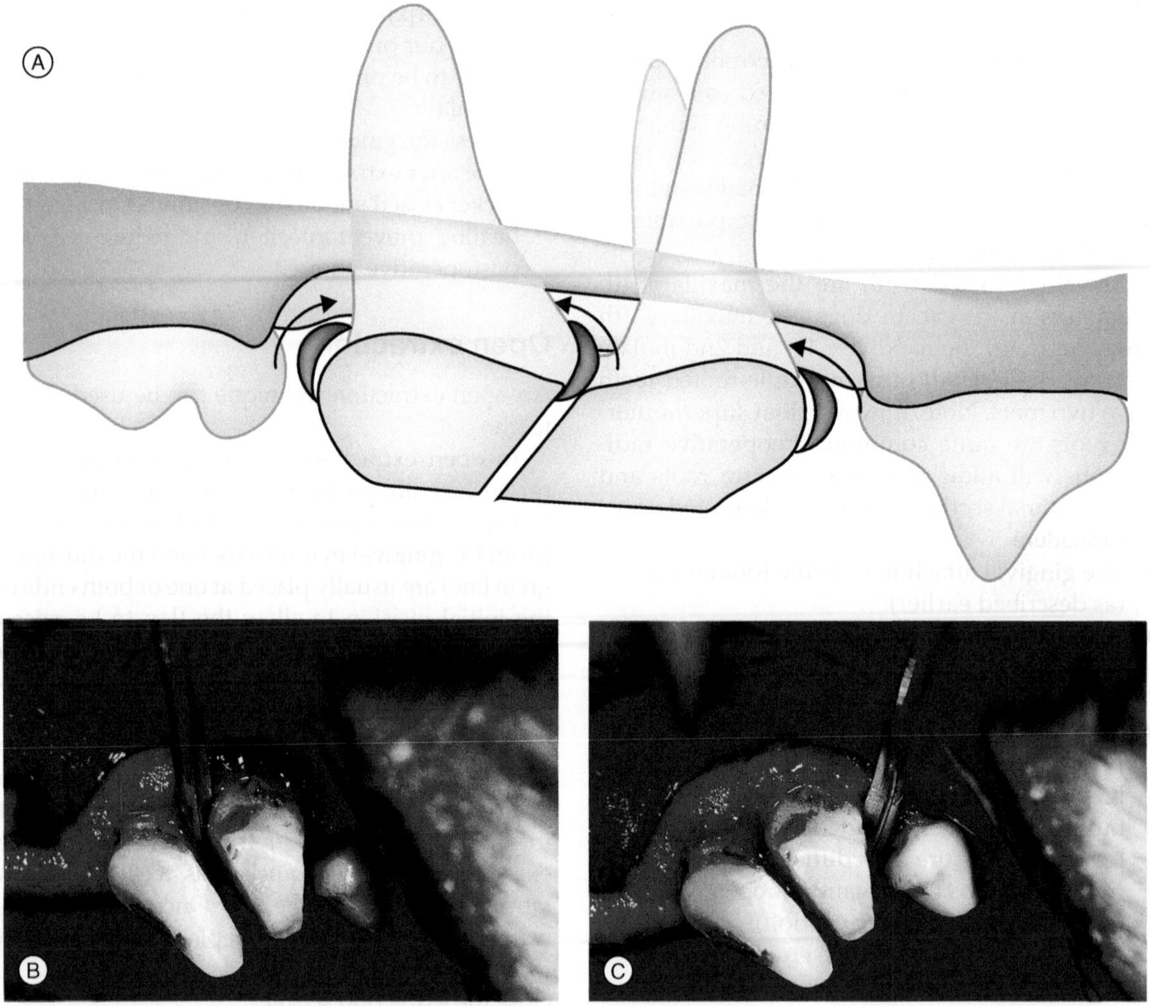

Fig. 11.4 **Using a dental elevator in a horizontal fashion.**
A: In addition to using the elevator in an apical direction, it can be inserted in a horizontal fashion between the tooth sections (shown in cross-section in the illustration) and rotated on its long axis to help tear periodontal fibres, so loosening the root. It can also be used mesially and distally, in which case, ensure that the alveolar margin is used as the fulcrum, not the adjacent tooth.
B: The elevator is inserted between the tooth sections and gently rotated.
C: The elevator inserted distally. Note that the alveolar bone is used as the fulcrum, i.e. not the mesial surface of the 1st molar, to prevent iatrogenic loosening of the molar!

- Short releasing incisions (extending from the gingival margin to just beyond the mucogingival line) are placed at the rostral and distal ends of the initial incision. Some clinicians prefer a long distal releasing incision (Fig. 11.6A)
- Periosteal elevators are used to lift the gingiva and mucosa from the bone overlying the buccal aspect of the canine root (Figs 11.5B and 11.6B)
- The buccal bone plate overlying the root is drilled away. It is usually not necessary to remove bone to the apex, only to two-thirds of the root length (Figs 11.5C and 11.6C). A size 2 or 4 bur is best for cats, size 6 for dogs, and size 8 for giant breeds. Water-cooling of

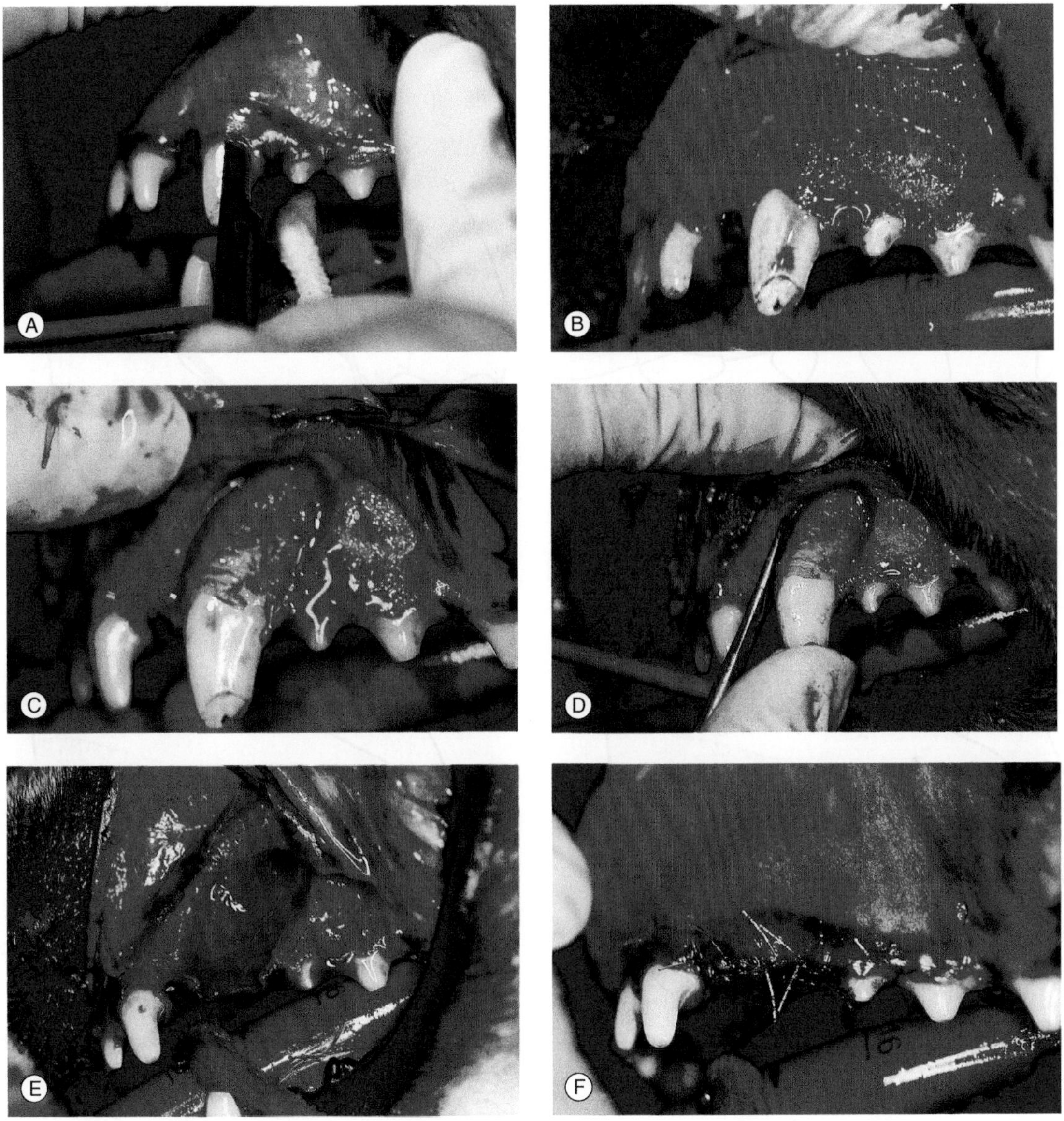

Fig. 11.5 Open extraction – maxillary canine (clinical slides).

A: Cutting the epithelial attachment.

B: A full thickness flap (extending from the gingival margin past the mucogingival junction) has been elevated to expose most of the buccal alveolar bone plate). Note the short mesial and distal releasing incisions.

C: Approximately two-thirds of the buccal bone plate overlying the root has been drilled away (a size 6 round bur in a high speed handpiece was used). The bone overlying the apical third of the root has not been removed. In addition, a gutter between the bone and tooth has been created on the mesial and distal aspects of the tooth.

D: An appropriately sized elevator placed in the mesial gutter. The instrument is rotated along its long axis. It is held in tension for 10–30 seconds at a time, alternating between mesial and distal until the tooth becomes loose. It is useful to use a luxator to cut the buccal apical periodontal fibres. Once the tooth is so loose that it can be moved freely in the socket, it can be gripped with fingers and lifted out.

E: Ensure that a clean coagulum forms in the socket.

F: The flap has been replaced and sutured to the palatal mucosa to close the extraction socket. There must be no tension on the suture line or the flap will break down!

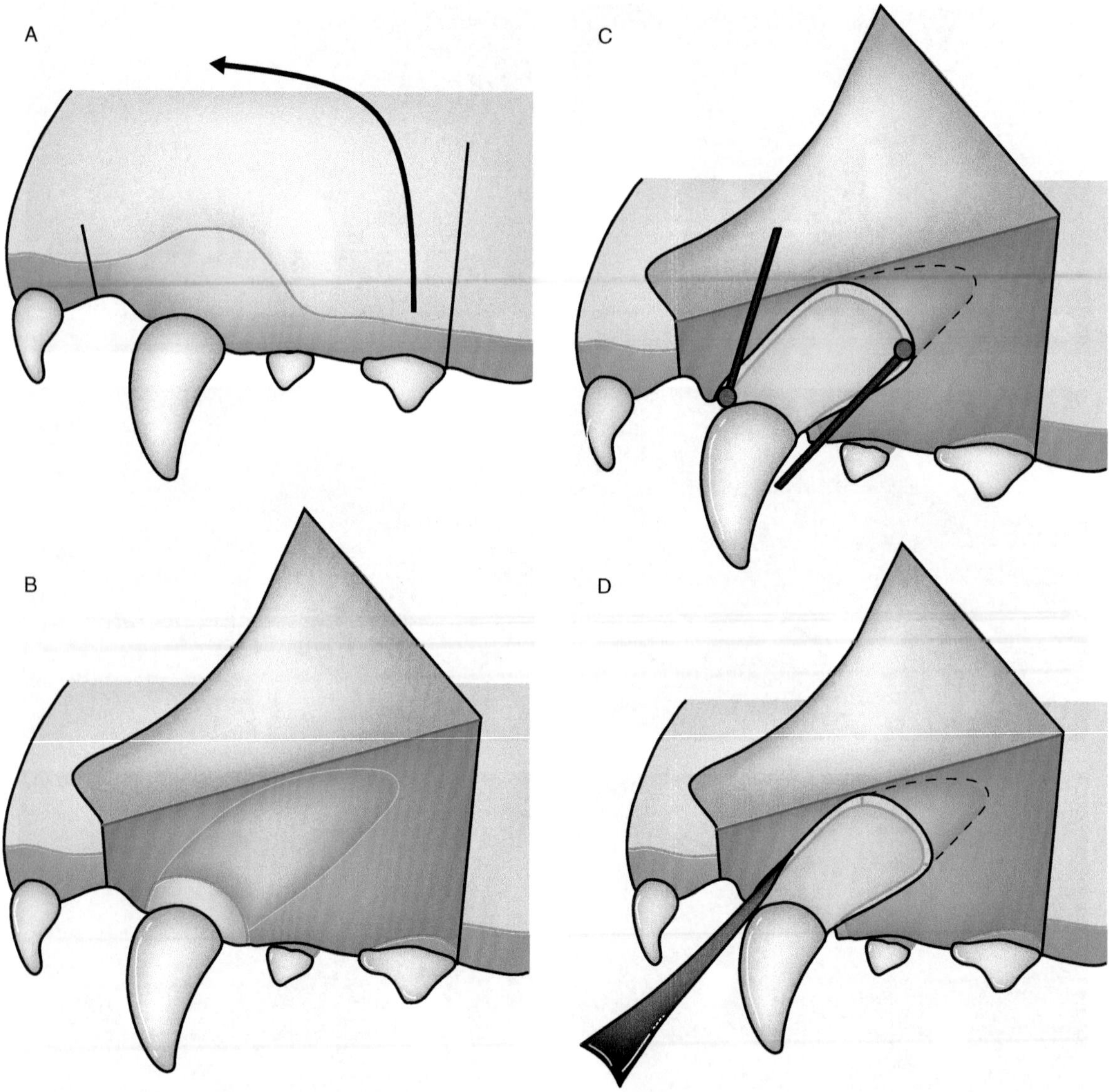

Fig. 11.6 Open extraction – maxillary canine (diagrammatic representation).
A: The primary incision and two releasing incisions have been placed.
B: The flap has been raised and reflected rostrally.
C: Buccal bone plate has been removed and the mesial and distal gutters between bone and tooth have been created.
D: Elevators are applied to rotate the tooth along its long axis to break the periodontal ligament fibres and loosen the tooth.
E: Sectional view of placement of the elevator in the gutter (G). Note the thin layer of bone on the nasal aspect of the maxillary canine alveolus.

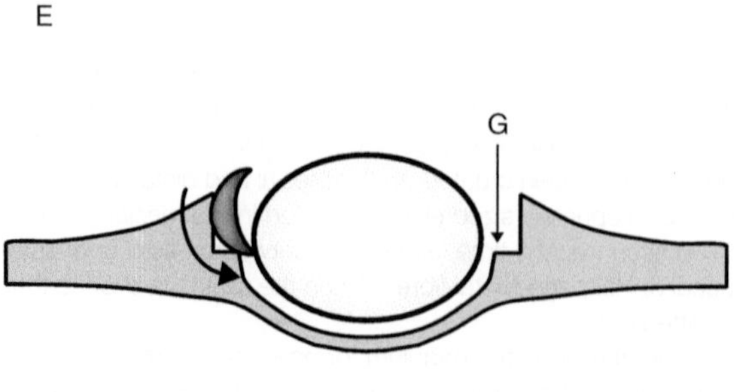

the bur is mandatory to avoid thermal damage to the bone
- The round bur is used to create a trough or gutter between the tooth root and the alveolar bone on the rostral and distal root surfaces (Figs 11.5C and 11.6C)
- An elevator of appropriate size is placed in one of the troughs and rotated along its long axis. This action will rotate the tooth along its long axis (Figs 11.5D and 11.6D). The aim is to break down the palatal periodontal fibres and those of the root tip, but avoid levering the root tip into the nasal cavity (Fig. 11.6E). The elevator is rotated to stretch the fibres, and held for 10–30 seconds at a time, repeating at each side until the tooth becomes loose, and can be easily removed. A luxator can be used to cut the buccal apical periodontal fibres
- A bur is used to smooth the edges of the alveolus. If the socket is filled with debris, it is gently flushed out prior to closure. For optimal healing, a clean clot should form in the socket (Fig. 11.5E)
- The flap is replaced and sutured *without tension* to the palatal mucosa to close the extraction socket. Simple interrupted sutures are used with an absorbable suture material with a swaged on needle (Fig. 11.5F)

Mandibular canine

Extraction of a periodontally sound mandibular canine is difficult. This tooth can be extracted using either a buccal or lingual approach. If using a buccal approach, be careful to avoid damage to the neurovascular bundle exiting the mental foramina while raising the flap. A lingual approach is possible, but gives poor visualisation.

My preferred method is a combined buccal and lingual approach as follows:

- The buccal flap is raised in a similar fashion to that described for the maxillary canine. The large neurovascular bundle exiting at one of the mental foramina (usually the middle foramen) must not be transected. It is visualised and carefully dissected free so it can be reflected together with the flap
- A gingival flap is also raised on the lingual aspect of the tooth
- Approximately 30% of the buccal alveolar bone plate is drilled away. The bone is removed to a level just apical to where the root is at its widest
- The crown is amputated just above the cemento-enamel junction (round or fissure bur) to allow easier access to the lingual surface
- Approximately 20% of the lingual alveolar bone plate is drilled away. Ensure that the flap is protected from the bur
- Mesial and distal gutters between tooth root and bone are created as described for the maxillary canine
- To loosen the tooth, elevators are used in the buccal mesial and distal gutters as described for extraction of the maxillary canine. In addition, luxators should be used to cut the buccal apical periodontal fibres. On the lingual aspect, luxators are used to cut periodontal ligament fibres and create enough space for elevators of increasing size to be used
- It may be necessary to remove additional alveolar bone, especially lingually. Try to maintain as much of the alveolar bone as possible to preserve the strength of the mandible
- Close the defect by suturing the buccal flap to the palatal flap. There must be no tension on the suture line

Maxillary 4th premolars and maxillary and mandibular molars in the dog

These teeth, if periodontally compromised, can be removed by sectioning, and closed extraction. If the teeth are periodontally sound, open extraction is recommended.

Primary teeth

Primary teeth can be extracted using either a closed or open technique. Preoperative radiographs are mandatory to give information as to the position and extent of primary tooth root resorption and the location and stage of development of the adjacent permanent tooth.

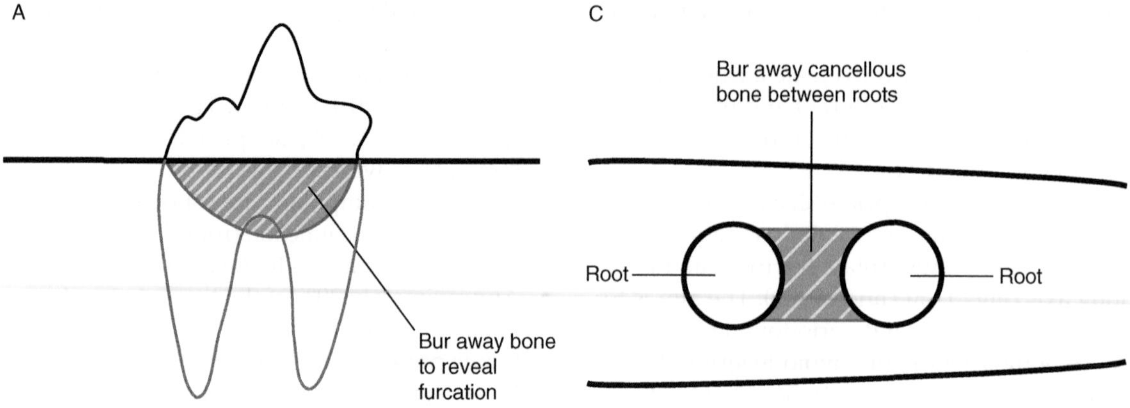

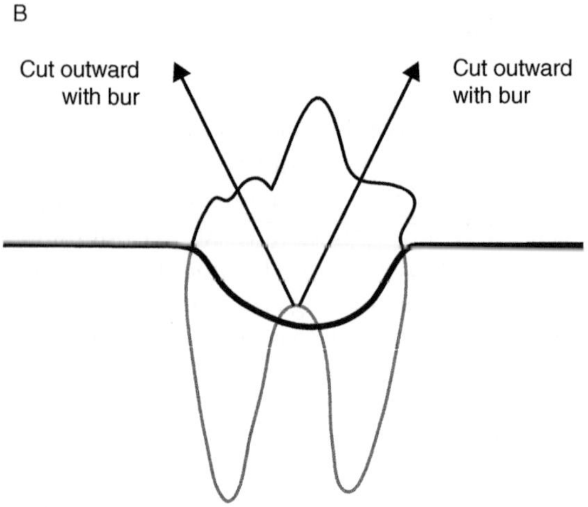

Fig. 11.7 Extraction of a feline lower molar.
A: After raising the gingival flaps, bur away shaded area of bone. Remove enough of the buccal alveolar bone plate to clearly expose the furcation.
B: Make two cuts from the furcation, at 45°, one rostrally and one distally, and drill from the furcation towards the occlusal surface of the crown. These cuts section the tooth into two single-rooted units and remove the bulk of the crown.
C: (View looking down on mandible). Bur away the cancellous bone between the two roots. The depth should be the same as the root length. Be careful not to enter the mandibular canal.

The extraction procedure is the same as for permanent teeth but care must be used to avoid damage to adjacent developing permanent dentition.

Special considerations with feline teeth

The most common diseases necessitating tooth extraction in cats are odontoclastic resorptive lesions (ORL), periodontitis and traumatic dental injuries resulting in pulpal exposure.

Small single-rooted teeth

In the cat, the incisors, the maxillary 2nd premolar and the maxillary molar are small single-rooted teeth. They can generally be removed using a closed technique. The technique is the same as already described in the 'Closed extraction' section, but a gentle approach should be used.

Canine teeth

The canine teeth, unless affected by severe periodontitis, require an open extraction technique as already described in the 'Open extraction' section.

Multiple-rooted teeth

In the cat, these are the maxillary and mandibular 3rd and 4th premolars and the mandibular molar. These teeth are every veterinary surgeon's nightmare due to the ease with which they fracture during extraction. This leaves roots, with or without pieces of crown attached, which must be removed. Although it might be tempting to leave these roots and hope they will resorb, or that the gingiva will grow over them, this is negligent. Every attempt should be made to retrieve such root remnants. If this is not technically possible, the owner must be informed that extraction was incomplete. Postoperative clinical and radiographic monitoring is mandatory. While some root remnants may resorb, others may result in inflammatory disease. If inflammatory disease occurs, then the root remnants must be extracted.

Multiple-rooted teeth in the cat can be removed using either a closed or open technique. The closed technique is identical to that already described above, but gentle technique is essential. In addition, ensure selection of appropriately sized instruments to avoid iatrogenic root fracture. Open extraction in the cat is similar to that already described above, but with the modifications suggested in the next paragraph.

A modified technique for extracting multirooted teeth in cats is proposed. The aim of the modification is to simplify removal and preserve alveolar bone. In the following, it is described for the mandibular teeth. The method can be adapted for removal of the maxillary multirooted teeth.

- Raise a gingival flap both buccally and lingually
- Remove enough alveolar bone to expose the furcation (Fig. 11.7A)
- A small round bur, usually size 2, is used to make two cuts from the furcation, at 45°, one distally and one mesially (Fig. 11.7B). These cuts will remove the bulk of the crown, leaving only a small point of crown on each individual root
- Use either a size 2 or size 4 round bur to remove the cancellous bone between the two roots. The depth should be the same as the root length, but not long enough to enter the mandibular canal (Fig. 11.7C). If in doubt, measure the distance on your radiographs
- Each root is then only supported by bone on three sides, a small luxator or elevator can be eased into the space created by the bur, and the roots can be loosened and removed
- If necessary, remove additional buccal bone
- Remove any sharp bony edges
- Suture the buccal flap to the lingual flap without tension

Summary

- Tooth extraction is the remit of the veterinary surgeon
- Extraction of teeth is a surgical procedure. There are two basic types of extraction – simple (closed) and surgical (open) techniques
- Tooth extraction demands suitable equipment, instrumentation and surgical technical skills if patient morbidity is to be minimised
- A good light source is essential – good visibility simplifies the procedure greatly
- It is necessary to be aware of possible complications so that any equipment, materials or medications can be available immediately
- Extraction is performed under radiographic control including, in problem cases, intraoperative X-rays

FURTHER READING

Emily, P. & Penman, S. (1994) Extraction and oronasal fistula closure. *Handbook of Small Animal Dentistry*, 2nd edn. London: Pergamon Press, Ch. 8, pp. 95–106.

Gorrel, C. & Robinson, J. (1995) Periodontal therapy and extraction technique. In: Crossley, D.A. & Penman, S. (eds) *Manual of Small Animal Dentistry*. Cheltenham: BSAVA, Ch. 14, pp. 139–149.

Holmstrom, S., Frost, P. & Eisner, E. (1988) Exodontics. *Veterinary Dental Techniques*. Philadelphia: WB Saunders, Ch. 6, pp. 215–254.

Mulligan, T., Aller, M. & Williams, C. (1998) *Atlas of Canine and Feline Dental Radiography*. Trenton, NJ: Veterinary Learning Systems.

12

Dental diseases in lagomorphs and rodents

With Leen Verhaert

Lagomorphs and rodents are increasingly popular pets. These 'pocket pets' have a high incidence of oral/dental problems. Most of the problems are related to the anatomical peculiarities of their dentition in combination with poor husbandry, i.e. feeding a non-abrasive diet resulting in abnormal wear and malocclusion.

While there are many similarities between lagomorphs and rodents with regard to type of dentition, oral/dental conditions and treatment options, there are also significant differences. In addition, there are differences within the rodent group.

This chapter will describe the normal anatomy of the dentition and the common oral/dental conditions of lagomorphs and rodents.

TYPES OF TEETH

There are two basic types of teeth:

- brachyodont
- hypsodont.

The brachyodont tooth has a short crown : root ratio, with a true root. Once the tooth has matured, the root apex closes and the potential for further tooth growth ceases. Humans, dogs, cats and ferrets have a brachyodont dentition.

The hypsodont tooth is a tooth with a long crown, and a comparatively short root. The subgingival part of the crown is called the reserve crown. Hypsodont teeth are either radicular or aradicular. The radicular hypsodont tooth eventually forms a true root. The tooth grows for most of the life of the animal, but late in life the root apex closes and tooth growth ceases. Horses and cows have radicular hypsodont teeth. The aradicular hypsodont tooth never forms a true root with an apex and the tooth grows continuously throughout the animal's life. Rabbits, guinea pigs and chinchillas have aradicular hypsodont teeth. The incisors of all rodents are aradicular hypsodont, while the cheek teeth are either aradicular hypsodont or brachyodont depending on the species.

If eruption of continuously growing teeth is hindered, e.g. mechanical obstruction due to a malocclusion resulting in abnormal occlusal forces, the continued growth of the tooth will result in destruction of the alveolar bone and apparent 'apical growth' of the tooth. This may result in perforation of the cortical bone.

DENTAL ANATOMY

Lagomorphs

The order Lagomorpha includes rabbits, hares, cottontails and pikas. All teeth in lagomorphs are aradicular hypsodont. They have four incisor teeth in the upper jaw. This clearly differentiates them from rodents, who only have two incisors in the upper jaw. The lagomorphs do not have canine teeth.

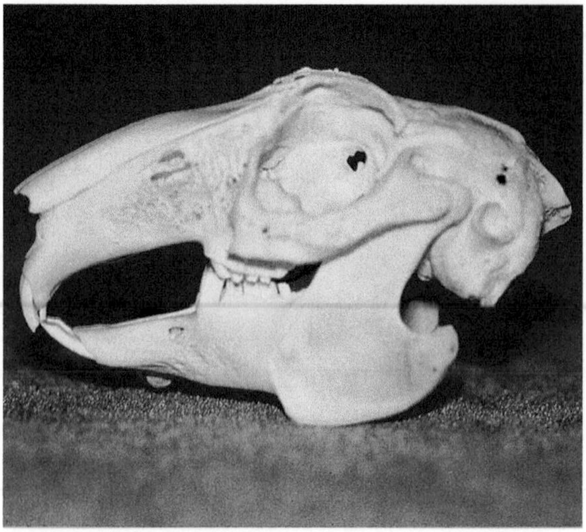

Fig. 12.1 Normal – rabbit skull. At rest, the incisors are held in occlusion and the cheek teeth are out of occlusion.

Lagomorph dental formula
2 × { I 2/1 : C 0/0 : P 3/2 : M 3/3 }

The four incisor teeth in the upper jaw are placed in two rows with the two large incisors located labially, and the two smaller rudimentary incisors (peg teeth) located palatally. In occlusion, the crown tips of the mandibular incisor teeth rest between the first and second row of upper jaw incisors. At rest, the incisors are held in occlusion and the cheek teeth are held out of occlusion (Crossley, 1995a). A relatively normal rabbit skull is depicted in Figure 12.1.

Rabbits do not gnaw like rodents, unless there is some cheek tooth problem interfering with normal mastication (Crossley, 1995a). The incisors are mainly used in a lateral slicing motion, to cut food into smaller pieces. The large upper incisors grow at an average rate of 2.0 mm per week and the lower incisors at a rate of 2.4 mm per week (Wiggs & Lobprise, 1995). A rabbit with normal incisor occlusion, eating a normally abrasive diet such as hay, grass and fresh greens, will wear down the teeth at a similar rate. The incisor teeth have thick white enamel on the labial surface and almost no enamel on the palatal/lingual surface. Normal tooth wear thus results in a chisel-shaped tooth as the softer dentine wears down faster than the thick enamel. A large diastema separates the incisor teeth from the premolar and molar teeth (cheek teeth).

The upper jaw is wider than the mandible (anisognathic) and when there are no cheek tooth problems, and no other interference such as overgrown incisors, the rabbit chews its foods using a wide lateral (side to side) motion.

Rodents

Rodentia is the largest mammal order, with weights ranging from 4 g to over 50 kg. All rodents are 'gnawers', with a wide rostrocaudal movement range in the temporomandibular joint and chisel-shaped continuously growing incisor teeth designed for this dorsoventral motion. They are anisognathic, but in contrast to the lagomorphs, the mandible is wider than the maxilla.

While the incisors are aradicular hypsodont, the cheek teeth are either aradicular hypsodont or brachyodont depending on species. The strict herbivores eating a highly abrasive diet have aradicular hypsodont cheek teeth, e.g. guinea pig and chinchilla. Species eating less abrasive diets, e.g. mice, rats and hamsters, have brachyodont cheek teeth.

The dental formula varies among the species, ranging from 16 to 22 teeth. However, all rodents have four incisors (one in each quadrant) and no canine teeth. A diastema separates the incisors from the cheek teeth.

Rodent dental formulae
Guinea pig and chinchilla: 2 × { I 1/1 : C 0/0 : P 1/1 : M 3/3 } Rat, mouse, gerbil: 2 × { I 1/1 : C 0/0 : P 0/0 : M 3/3 } Hamster: 2 × { I 1/1 : C 0/0 : P 0/0 : M 2-3/2-3 }

At rest (Fig. 12.2A), the mandible is in a caudal position and the incisors are out of occlusion (Crossley, 1995b). During gnawing, the incisors are held in occlusion (Fig. 12.2B).

As in lagomorphs, the enamel layer of the incisors is thickest on the labial surface, with almost none present at the palatal/lingual aspect, resulting

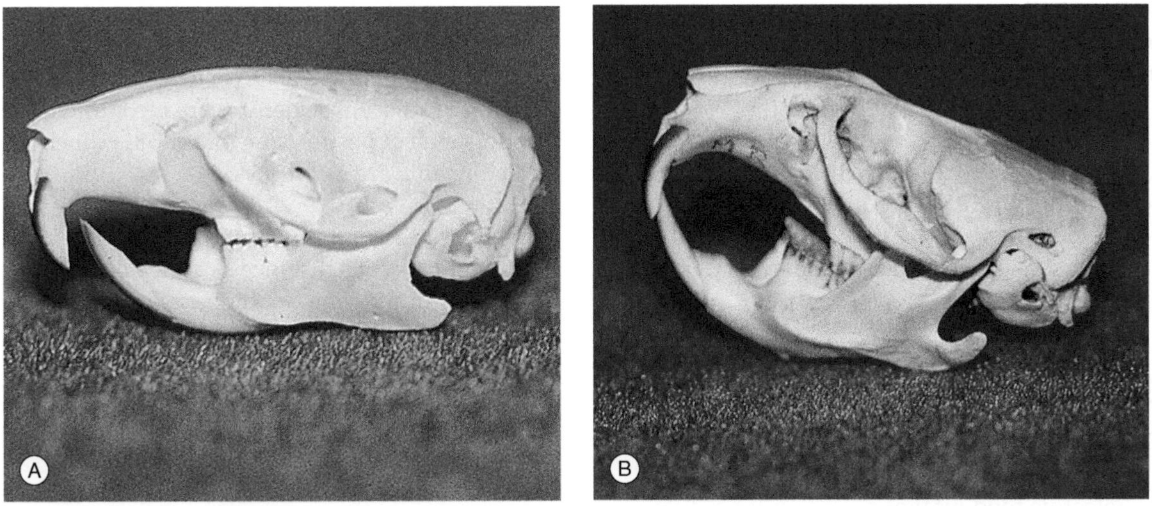

Fig. 12.2 Normal – rat skull.
A: At rest, the mandible is held in a caudal position. The incisors are then out of occlusion and the cheek teeth are in occlusion.
B: For gnawing, the mandible is moved rostrally so that the incisor teeth are brought into occlusion.

in a chisel-shaped pattern of tooth wear. The enamel is usually orange-yellow in colour. However, the guinea pig has white enamel.

HUSBANDRY

Tooth overgrowth is by far the most common dental problem in rabbits. While incisor overgrowth due to an inherited skeletal malocclusion does occur, the most common cause of tooth overgrowth is insufficient wear of the continuously growing teeth caused by feeding a non-abrasive diet, e.g. dry pellets only. The affected animal is often presented late in the process. In many cases the patient is presented when disease is too advanced to be amenable to intervention, and euthanasia is required for a condition that could have been prevented.

Weekly weighing of every pocket pet is strongly recommended. Weight loss always requires investigation. Disease may thus be identified and treatment instituted earlier.

The ideal diet for the strictly herbivorous pocket pets consists of grass and coarse hay as the main components. This may be supplemented with fresh vegetables and dry pellets. If dry pellets are fed, they should only form a maximum of 10% of the total diet. A diet such as this will not only help in preventing overgrowth of the teeth, but is also healthier for the gastrointestinal system. All rodents need material to gnaw on.

Guinea pigs need vitamin C supplementation (Flecknell, 1991; Schaeffer & Donnelly, 1997). A daily dose of 10 mg/kg is recommended for normal activity; this should be increased (up to 30 mg/kg) in situations of stress (e.g. change of environment, pregnancy, illness, new pet). There are commercially available vitamin C drops that can be added to the food or the water. Alternatively, human vitamin C tablets can be crushed and mixed with the diet or the water. Vitamin C is unstable (easily oxidised by light and air); therefore, water solutions need to be changed daily.

Consequences of tooth overgrowth

Tooth overgrowth commonly results in malocclusion. Complications to malocclusion include:

- Traumatisation of oral soft tissues (cheeks, tongue) by the overgrown teeth
- Apical overgrowth with resultant penetration of upper teeth into the ocular sockets and/or sinuses
- Apical overgrowth of the mandibular teeth with resultant penetration of the ventral border of the alveolar bone

- Retrobulbar and/or facial abscessation
- Inability to close the mouth
- Inability to chew (lateral slicing motion in lagomorphs; gnawing in rodents)

With advanced disease, the animal is unable to eat and weight loss occurs. The oral discomfort is often associated with excessive salivation ('slobbers'), which predisposes to moist dermatitis (wet dewlap).

SIGNS OF DENTAL DISEASE

Signs that may be due to dental disease include:

- Selective food intake
- Dropping food from mouth
- Anorexia
- Ocular discharge
- Nasal discharge
- Continuous tooth grinding
- Excessive salivation
- Changes in grooming behaviour
- Accumulation of caecotrophs around the anus (predisposing to 'fly strike')

It must be emphasised that the above signs can occur with other disease processes. Anorexia is a very common sign of advanced oral disease, but it is also a sign of almost any disease in these animals. Lagomorphs and rodents affected by pain usually stop eating. Tooth grinding is more commonly associated with abdominal discomfort than with oral/dental disease.

Since animals with oral/dental disease are presented late in the disease process, they are often emaciated, dehydrated and obstipated. In addition, they are usually severely stressed from chronic discomfort/pain.

RADIOGRAPHIC EXAMINATION

Pocket pets presenting with signs of dental disease require radiographic evaluation.

Three basic skull views need to be taken, namely lateral, dorsoventral and rostrocaudal. Of these, the lateral view is usually the most informative. Additional oblique lateral views may be necessary for some patients. When possible, additional intraoral views to avoid superimposition of adjacent structures are recommended.

Suggested exposure time for rabbit, guinea pig and chinchilla are as follows:

- Standard radiography unit: 15 mA and 75 kV, 50 cm film–focus distance as a starting point. For rostrocaudal views, higher exposure will be needed
- Dental radiography unit: exposure time comparable to exposure time for radiography of canine teeth in a medium to large breed dog (depending on the size of the animal)

Even with radiographic examination, a lot of the pathology will be missed. Radiographic interpretation by an experienced examiner will only reveal around 85% of the pathology present (Crossley, 2000). Computed tomographic (CT) scan will give more information, especially for the detection of early cheek tooth pathology (Crossley et al, 1998).

RABBITS

The healthy mouth

Incisor teeth

- The maxillary incisors have vertical grooves on the labial surfaces
- Held in occlusion at rest (with the crown tips of the mandibular incisors resting between the first and second row of maxillary incisors)
- Occlusal plane is horizontal
- Have chisel-shaped wear pattern

Cheek teeth

- The maxillary cheek teeth should be worn almost level with the gingiva
- The mandibular cheek teeth show only a few millimetres of crown (depending on the size of the rabbit)
- The occlusal plane is almost horizontal (10°)
- No spikes on any of the teeth

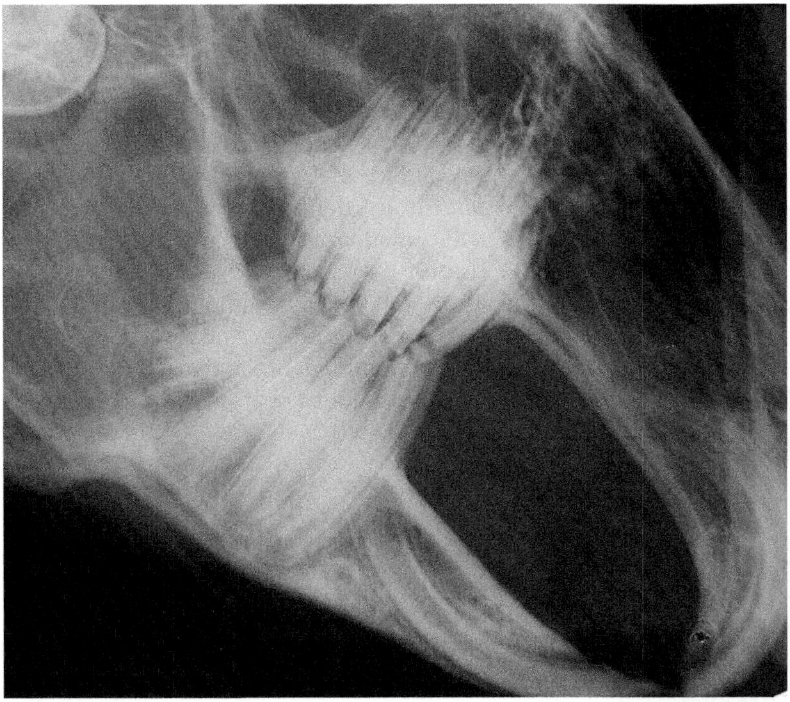

Fig. 12.3 Lateral radiograph of a normal rabbit. Note that the palatine shelf and the dorsal border of the mandible converge rostrally.

Normal radiographic features

Lateral view (Fig. 12.3)

- The palatine shelf and the dorsal border of the mandible converge rostrally
- Ideally, with the incisors in occlusion, the cheek teeth should be out of occlusion. This is rarely seen in pet rabbits. As soon as both are in occlusion, there is some degree of cheek tooth overgrowth. However, as long as the maxilla and mandible converge rostrally, this is not a clinical problem
- Smooth ventral mandibular border
- Normal radiolucencies of the periapical germinal tissues
- The apices of the maxillary incisor teeth should not penetrate the palatine shelf

Rostrocaudal view

- Occlusal plane: almost horizontal
- No spikes visible
- No tipping of teeth

Dorsoventral view

- Smooth bony contours, with only the lachrymal processes sticking out
- Orbits clear with smooth borders

The dorsoventral view does not usually contribute much extra information in the rabbit and we often omit it.

Incisor overgrowth

Incisor overgrowth is common in rabbits. The condition can be classified as primary or secondary depending on its cause. Primary incisor overgrowth is the consequence of an inherited skeletal malocclusion (maxillary brachygnathism resulting in a relative mandibular prognathism) and thus occurs early in life (within the first year). In contrast, secondary incisor overgrowth is the consequence of cheek tooth overgrowth and thus develops later in life (adult, usually more than a year old). Most rabbits presented for treatment of incisor overgrowth do not have an inherited

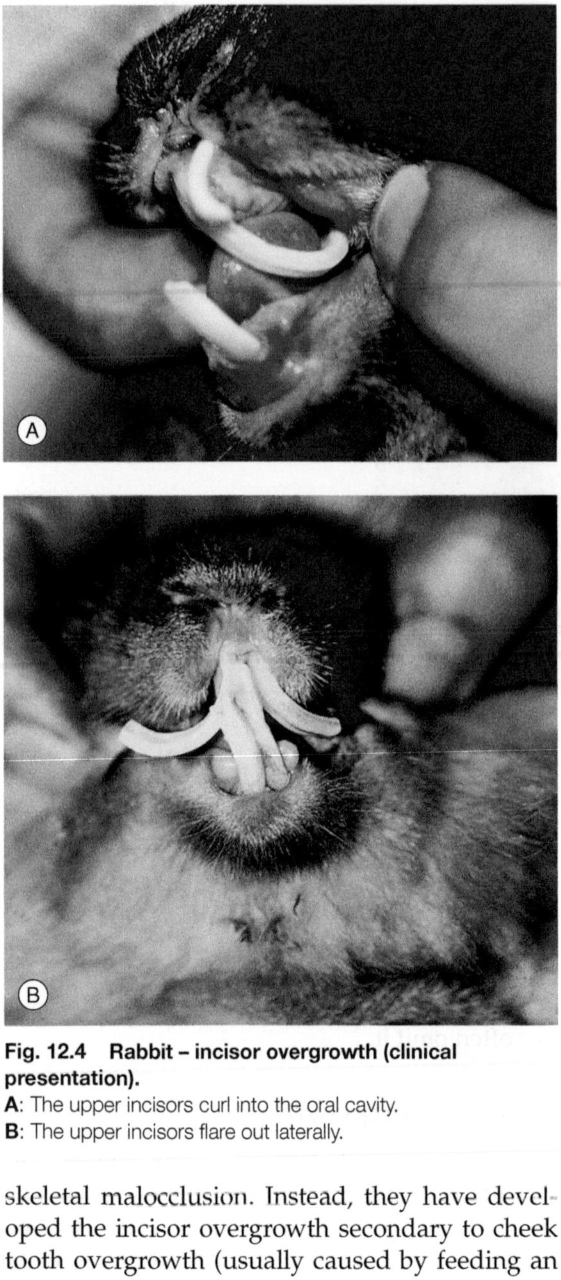

Fig. 12.4 Rabbit – incisor overgrowth (clinical presentation).
A: The upper incisors curl into the oral cavity.
B: The upper incisors flare out laterally.

skeletal malocclusion. Instead, they have developed the incisor overgrowth secondary to cheek tooth overgrowth (usually caused by feeding an inappropriate diet).

Primary incisor overgrowth occurs regularly in dwarf rabbits. Due to the jaw length discrepancy (i.e. the mandible is too long with respect to the maxilla), normal incisor occlusion is not established. The mandibular incisors occlude either level with or rostral to the large labial row of maxillary incisors. The result is that normal incisor wear does not occur. The upper incisors may curl inward (Fig. 12.4A) or flare out laterally (Fig. 12.4B), and the mandibular incisors protrude from the mouth. If eruption of the maxillary incisors is hindered, e.g. mechanical obstruction by abnormal occlusal forces, then tooth growth will occur in an apical direction and may result in perforation of the palatine shelf. When significant incisor malocclusion has developed, the animal cannot close its mouth normally and secondary cheek tooth overgrowth will develop over time. If the condition is identified early, i.e. before excessive secondary cheek tooth overgrowth has occurred, the prognosis is relatively good with appropriate treatment.

Cheek tooth overgrowth

Cheek tooth abnormalities are very common in pet rabbits (Fig. 12.5). As already mentioned, most rabbits presented for treatment of incisor tooth overgrowth have the incisor overgrowth secondarily to the cheek tooth overgrowth, i.e. the cheek tooth overgrowth is the primary cause. Although calcium and vitamin D deficiency may be involved in the aetiology (Harcourt-Brown & Baker, 2001), the primary cause of cheek tooth overgrowth is thought to be feeding diets that provide insufficient abrasion (Crossley, 1995a; Redrobe, 1997).

Early cheek tooth overgrowth is not obvious without examination under general anaesthesia and radiography. The incisors may still be normally occluding and wearing. Consequently, animals with cheek tooth overgrowth are usually presented late in the disease process (Fig. 12.6). In fact, it is often when the animal is unable to close its mouth and secondary incisor overgrowth and malocclusion has occurred that treatment is sought. The owners assume that the problem is isolated to the incisor teeth. Client communication and education is essential.

Facial abscess

The development of facial abscesses is common in rabbits. They are usually associated with diseased teeth (Fig. 12.5), but may also occur due to

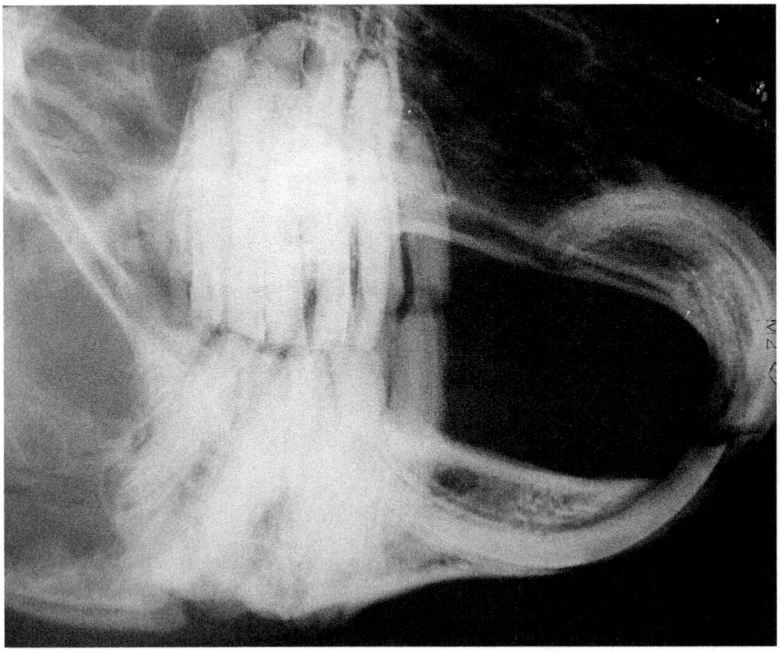

Fig. 12.5 Rabbit – severe tooth overgrowth and abscessation (lateral radiograph). This rabbit has extensive tooth overgrowth (cheek tooth and secondary incisor tooth). The palatine shelf and dorsal border of the mandible are parallel. The maxillary cheek teeth show gross root elongation with associated abscess formation. The upper incisors are almost penetrating the palatine shelf. Most of the roots of the mandibular cheek are resorbing. The lower incisors are also showing gross root elongation. Euthanasia is the most humane option for this animal.

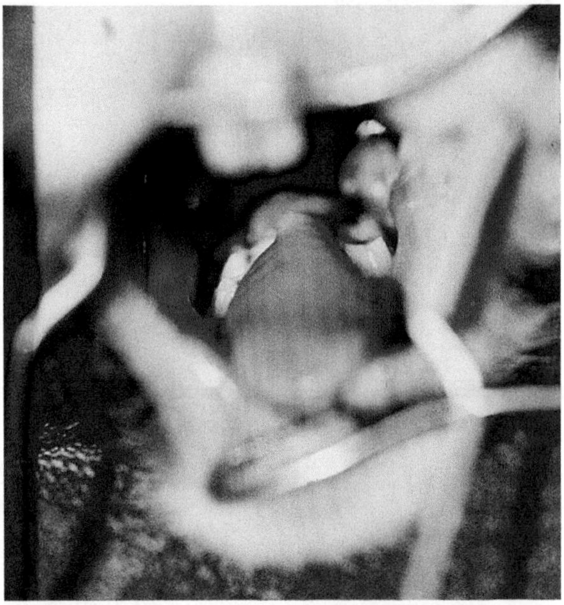

Fig. 12.6 Rabbit – cheek tooth overgrowth (clinical presentation). The mandibular cheek teeth are developing lingual spikes, which may traumatise the tongue.

mucosal perforation by overgrown teeth (dental spikes) or due to external wounds. While abscesses caused by mucosal trauma from spikes on overgrown teeth or external wounds are easy to treat, the abscesses arising due to dental pathology are more difficult to manage.

'Dental' abscesses can be of endodontic origin (pulpal disease) or periodontic origin. In the latter, foreign material (food) that is impacted into the periodontal ligament causes destruction of the periodontium, which may be so extensive that the endodontic system becomes involved secondarily. The lesions are often large at the time of diagnosis and the prognosis for complete cure is usually poor. In fact, euthanasia is often indicated.

Other dental conditions

Periodontal disease, i.e. plaque-induced inflammation of the periodontium, in rabbits is reportedly not as common as in the dog and cat (Wiggs & Lobprise, 1995). However, periodontal disease does occur and is often missed on clinical examination. The sulci of all teeth should be investigated with a periodontal probe. Treatment is similar to that for other species, i.e. professional cleaning and extraction of severely affected teeth. In the rabbit, loss of periodontal attachment is more often caused by food impaction triggering destruction of the periodontium rather than

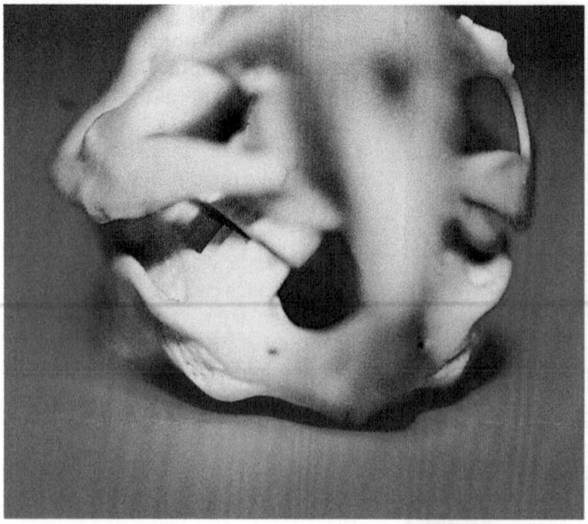

Fig. 12.7 Normal – guinea pig skull. The occlusal plane of the cheek teeth has a 30° angle.

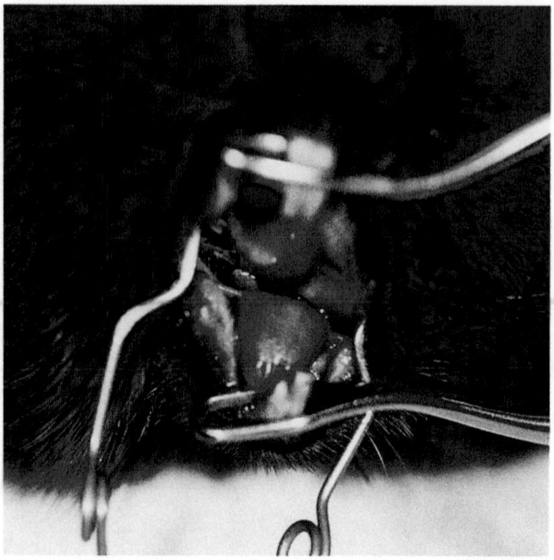

Fig. 12.8 Guinea pig – severe cheek tooth overgrowth (clinical presentation). The tongue is trapped by the overgrown mandibular cheek teeth.

irritation from plaque accumulation (Redrobe, 1997). Often the periodontal destruction is severe and spreads to involve the endodontic system, usually resulting in the formation of a periapical abscess. Once this complication has occurred, prognosis is poor and often warrants euthanasia of the affected animal.

Both caries and root resorption have been described in rabbits. When the lesions are small, they may wear away. Extensive lesions require extraction of the affected tooth or possibly restoration. The latter option requires referral to a specialist.

GUINEA PIGS

Guinea pigs are strictly herbivorous rodents, and have aradicular hypsodont cheek teeth.

The healthy mouth

- Incisor enamel is white in colour (in contrast to most other rodents)
- Incisors are worn down in a chisel-shaped pattern
- The occlusal plane of the incisors is horizontal
- At rest, the mandible is held in a caudal position and the incisor teeth are out of occlusion
- The mandible is wider than the maxilla

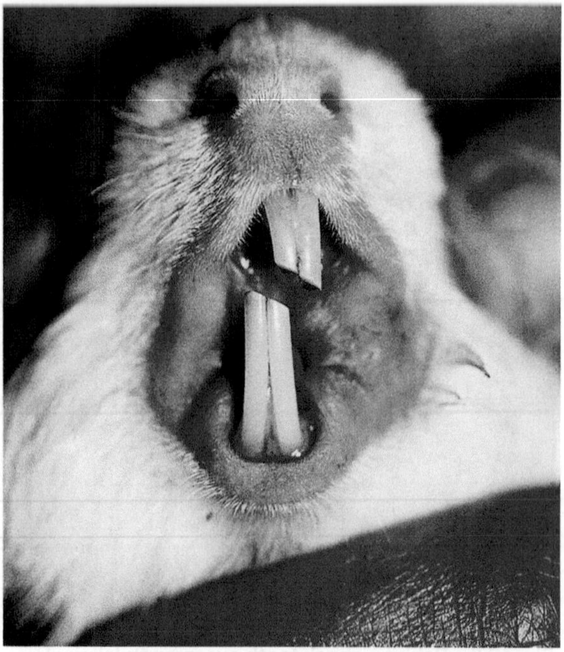

Fig. 12.9 Guinea pig – uneven wear of the incisor teeth (clinical presentation). The uneven wear of the incisor teeth was caused by overgrowth of the cheek teeth.

- The cheek teeth tip (the maxillary teeth buccally and the mandibular teeth lingually)
- The occlusal plane of the cheek teeth has a 30° angle (Fig. 12.7)

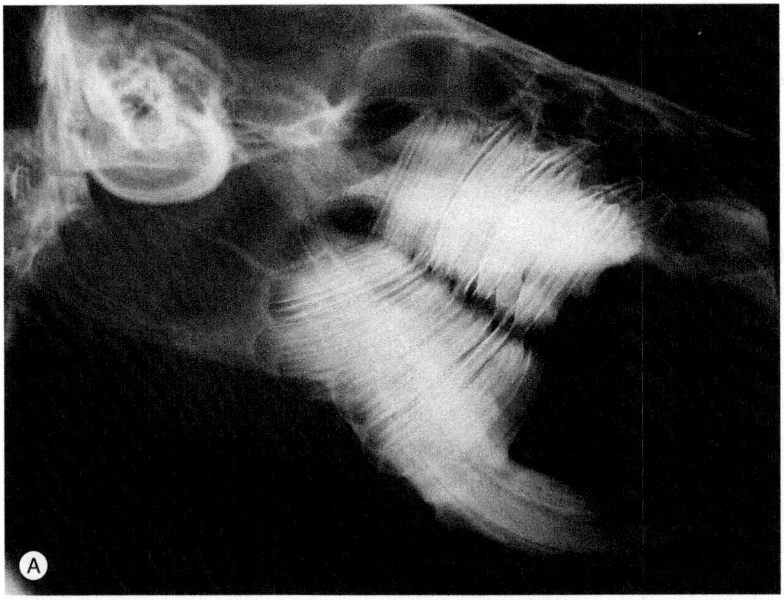

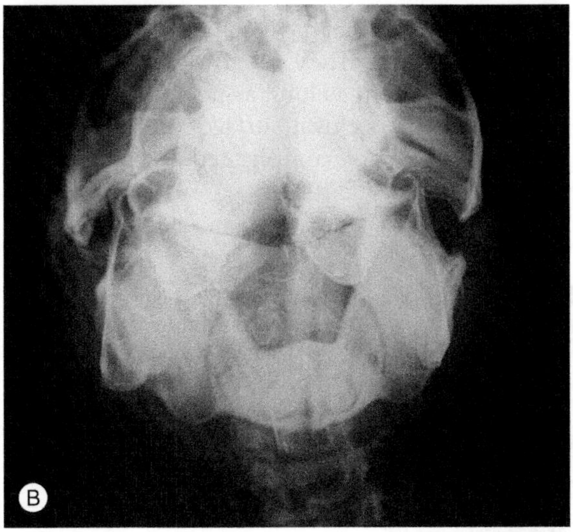

Fig. 12.10 Guinea pig – cheek tooth overgrowth (radiographic features).
A: Lateral view. The massive overgrowth of the cheek teeth is forcing the mouth open and the mandible is pushed rostrally.
B: Rostrocaudal view. This view is extremely helpful in guinea pigs. It allows visualisation of dental spikes and shows the tipping of the teeth.
Note also the nice image of the temporomandibular junction obtained with this view.

- The palatine shelf and dorsal border of the mandible converge rostrally
- The crowns of the cheek teeth are almost level with the gingiva

Incisor overgrowth

Primary incisor overgrowth is considered rare. When incisor overgrowth occurs, it is usually secondary to cheek tooth overgrowth. It may also be secondary to facial trauma.

Cheek tooth overgrowth

Most pet guinea pigs have some degree of cheek tooth overgrowth, and in many it will cause severe problems at some stage in life. The problems include:

- Tongue entrapment by the mandibular cheek teeth (Fig. 12.8)
- Lacerations of the buccal mucosa by dental spikes on the overgrown maxillary teeth
- Overgrowth, abnormal wear patterns and malocclusion of the incisor teeth (Fig. 12.9)
- Apical overgrowth of the cheek teeth with resultant perforation of the alveolar bone

The radiographic features of cheek tooth overgrowth in guinea pigs are shown in Figure 12.10A and B. In guinea pigs, the rostrocaudal view provides valuable information.

There is an association between cheek tooth overgrowth and hypovitaminosis C (Klaus & Bennett, 1999; Brown & Rosenthal, 1997a). The condition is often exacerbated by a vitamin C deficiency, which leads to collagen defects and resultant tipping of the teeth and/or eruption problems since collagen is necessary for anchoring the tooth in the socket (Schaeffer & Donnelly, 1997; Brown & Rosenthal, 1997a). Dental overgrowth in guinea pigs has also been linked with excessive selenium intake (Williams, 1976).

The animals are usually presented when pathology is advanced and prognosis is usually poor.

CHINCHILLAS

Chinchillas are herbivorous rodents, with aradicular hypsodont teeth. Dental disease is extremely common in this species; one report mentions 35% of apparently healthy chinchillas showing cheek tooth elongation on examination (Crossley, 2001a).

The healthy mouth

- Incisor enamel is orange-yellow in colour
- Incisors are worn down in a chisel-shaped pattern
- The occlusal plane of the incisors is horizontal
- At rest, the mandible is held in a caudal position, and the incisor teeth are out of occlusion
- The mandible is wider than the maxilla
- The cheek teeth are upright in position, i.e. do not tilt as in guinea pigs
- The cheek teeth have a horizontal occlusal plane
- The palatine shelf and dorsal border of the mandible converge rostrally
- The crowns of the cheek teeth are almost level with the gingiva

The radiographic features of a chinchilla with normal dentition and occlusion are depicted in Figure 12.11.

Incisor overgrowth

Primary incisor overgrowth is extremely rare. In a large survey (more than 700 animals were examined) investigating the incidence of dental disease in this species, only one animal with incisor overgrowth due to a maxillary brachygnathism was identified (Crossley, 2001). In contrast, secondary incisor overgrowth is common.

Cheek tooth overgrowth

Most pet chinchillas have some degree of cheek tooth elongation. They seem to cope well with simple elongation as long as no sharp spikes are formed on the occlusal surfaces, and as long as the process is not complicated by periodontal disease (Crossley, 2001).

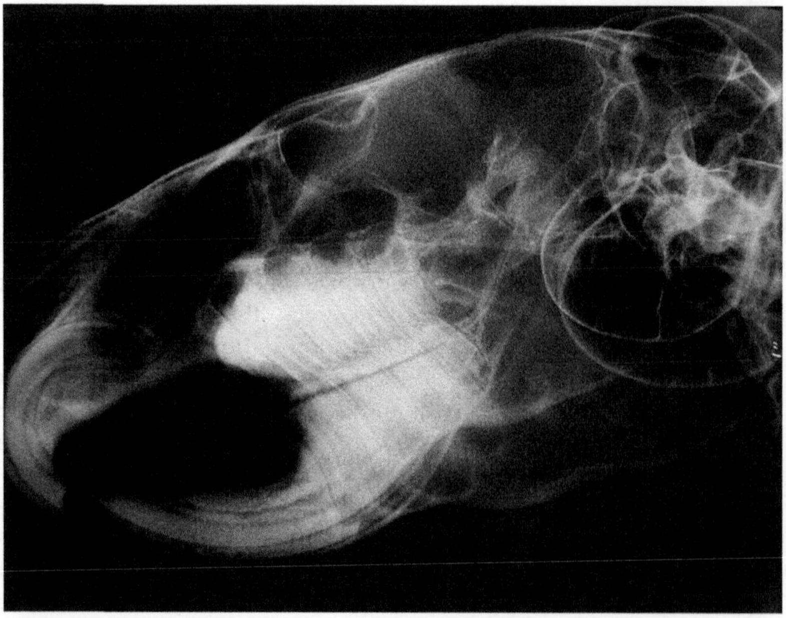

Fig. 12.11 Chinchilla – clinically healthy (radiographic features). The cheek teeth have short crowns and roots. The occlusal plane is smooth.

Due to the upright position of the cheek teeth, even slight overgrowth of the visible crown will result in occlusal forces that exceed eruptive forces. The visible crown will stop erupting. Instead, continued tooth growth will proceed in an apical direction (retrograde eruption) and result in apparent 'root' elongation. In the mandible, swellings associated with the apical growth of the check teeth are readily palpated along the ventro-lateral border even with minor overgrowth. This is a major difference between chinchillas and guinea pigs. Palpable swellings of the ventral mandibular border indicate early cheek tooth overgrowth in chinchillas. In guinea pigs, this clinical finding is evidence of advanced disease.

As cheek tooth overgrowth progresses, dramatic changes in the structure of the upper jaw and mandible occur (Figs 12.12 and 12.13). In the

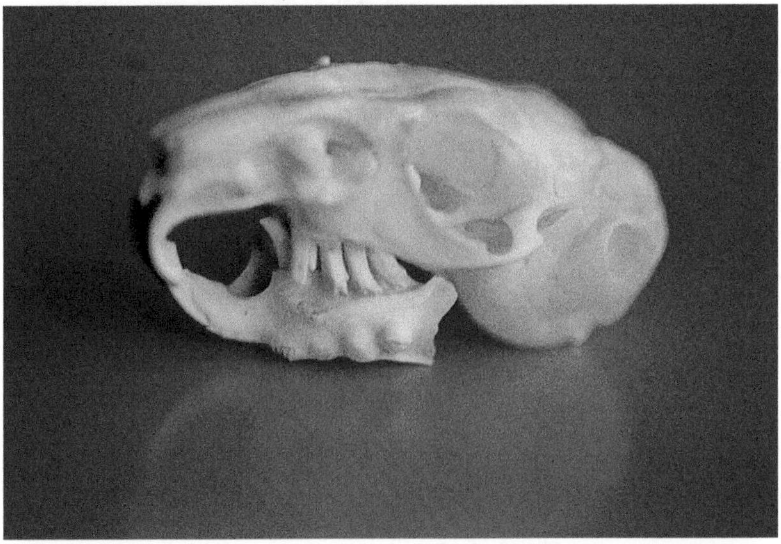

Fig. 12.12 Chinchilla skull – severe tooth overgrowth. This is a very advanced case.

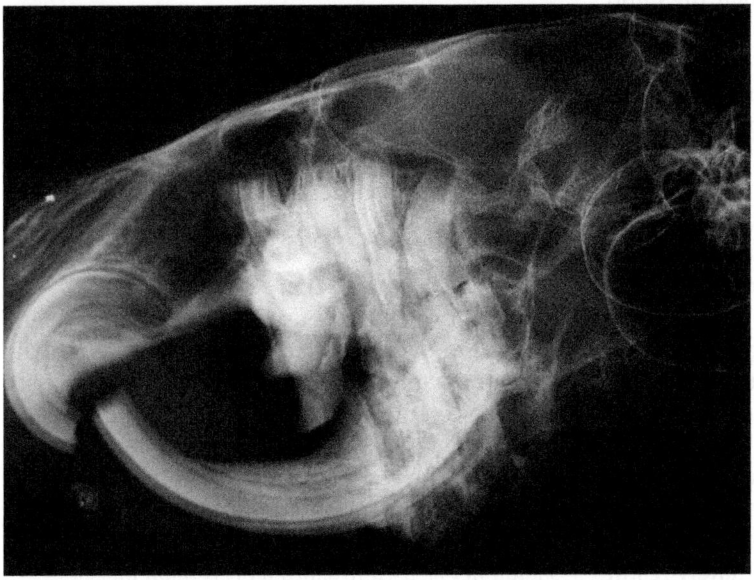

Fig. 12.13 Chinchilla – advanced cheek tooth pathology (lateral radiograph). Advanced cheek tooth problems. Note the root and crown elongation and the 'wavy' occlusal plane. Radical coronal reduction of the cheek teeth and change of feeding regimen resulted in clinical cure and weight gain. The same animal was re-presented two years later for recent weight loss because of dental disease that did not respond to treatment and he was euthanased.

upper jaw, the root elongation may present clinically as lachrymal overflow and/or eye protrusion. In the mandible, the cortical bone of the mandible may be destroyed during the root elongation, resulting in perforation. Since apical growth of the teeth occurs as an early response to overgrowth, pathology is usually advanced before there is obvious elongation of the visible crowns on intraoral clinical inspection.

Other dental conditions

Loss of periodontal attachment is more often caused by food impaction triggering destruction of the periodontium than by irritation from plaque accumulation.

Both caries and root resorption have been described in chinchillas (Crossley, 2001; Crossley et al, 1997). Starch and sugar are a significant proportion of the pet chinchilla's diet, and the diet is less abrasive than the diet in the wild. Therefore, incipient occlusal caries will not be worn down, as it would be in the wild animal.

RATS, MICE, HAMSTERS AND GERBILS

Rats, mice, hamsters and gerbils have brachyodont cheek teeth, sparing them from the severe malocclusion problems seen in guinea pigs and chinchillas.

Incisor overgrowth (Fig. 12.14) in these species is usually caused by lack of gnawing. They are usually fed a diet that requires minimal gnawing. Successful treatment is a combination of changing the diet and professional trimming of the teeth. These animals need to be presented with material to gnaw on, e.g. twigs of non-toxic trees such as fruit trees for the smaller species and whole nuts in the shell for the larger species.

Information in the literature regarding susceptibility of these species to plaque-induced periodontal disease is conflicting. While some authors report it to be relatively uncommon (Wiggs & Lobprise, 1995), others report it to be common in laboratory maintained animals (Miles & Crigson, 1990). In our experience, periodontal disease is common in pet rodents. This will ultimately result in exfoliation of the affected tooth. Treatment is the same as in other species, namely periodontal therapy and extraction of severely affected teeth.

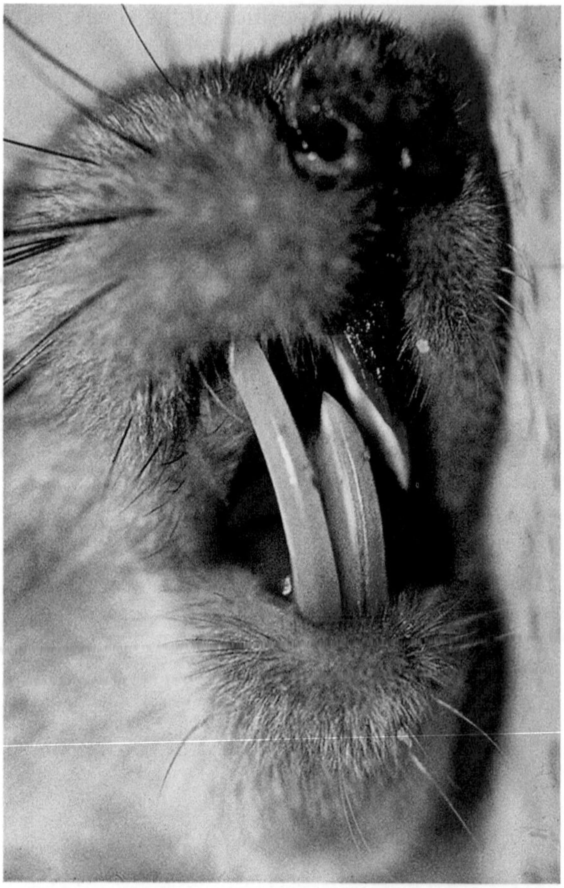

Fig. 12.14 Rat – incisor overgrowth (clinical presentation). Incisor overgrowth caused by lack of wear. One of the upper incisors is fractured.

TRAUMATIC TOOTH INJURIES

The most common cause of 'traumatic tooth injury' is probably the use of nail cutters (clippers) to shorten overgrown incisors. Apart from being an unpleasant procedure for the pet, the nail cutters shatter the tooth. The fracture may extend below the gingival margin and the pulp is often exposed. The resultant pulpal inflammation may be so severe that periapical abscessation develops and extensive treatment is required. *Nail cutters should not be used to shorten overgrown incisors.*

While the most common cause of tooth injury may be iatrogenic, all the pocket pets are prone to traumatic injuries. They are often kept for small children who do not handle them as carefully as one might like. In fact, accidentally dropping the pet to the floor is common. This type of trauma often results in tooth fracture (usually incisors), sometimes accompanied by jaw fracture.

TOOTH TRIMMING

Tooth trimming is the most commonly indicated procedure in lagomorph and rodent dentistry. The aim is to recreate normal, or near normal, occlusion. Improved husbandry, i.e. feeding an appropriately abrasive diet, will then help maintain normal occlusion as normal wear occurs.

Tooth trimming is a difficult and time-consuming procedure. It should be performed under general anaesthesia. While trimming incisors without general anaesthesia is possible, it is impossible to check and trim cheek teeth. The whole occlusion needs evaluation. It is rare that just the incisors need shaping. In fact, it is more common that the cause of the problem rests with the cheek tooth occlusion.

Equipment and instrumentation requirements (Figs 12.15 and 12.16) include:

- Good lighting
- Mouth gag
- Cheek dilator(s)
- Spatulas for protection of soft tissues
- Slow-speed straight handpiece
- High-speed handpiece
- Selection of slow-speed burs (straight handpiece fissure and acrylic burs of different sizes)
- Selection of high-speed burs (fissure and possible pear-shaped of different sizes)

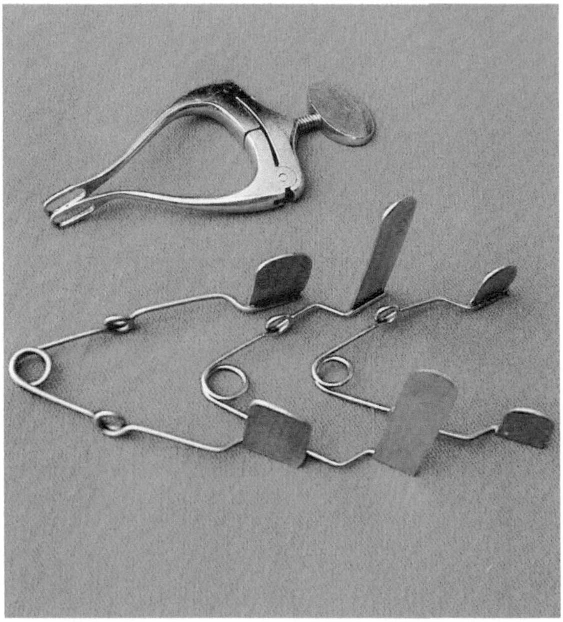

Fig. 12.15 Equipment 1 – gags and dilators.

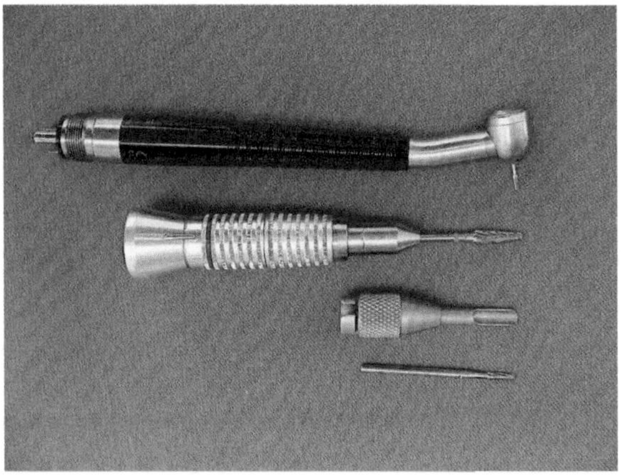

Fig. 12.16 Equipment 2 – burs and handpieces. From top to bottom: high-speed handpiece with friction grip fissure bur, straight low-speed handpiece with acrylic bur, protector for straight handpiece (HP) fissure bur, HP fissure bur.

EXTRACTION

Teeth affected by severe disease need extraction. In the pocket pets, there are rarely alternative treatments. Moreover, extraction may be preferable to trimming every few weeks. Specialised instrumentation is needed (Fig. 12.17), and with the increasing importance of rabbits and rodents as pets, these instruments are now available (e.g. Crossley luxator). For very small animals, instruments may need to be custom-made by bending hypodermic needles of suitable size.

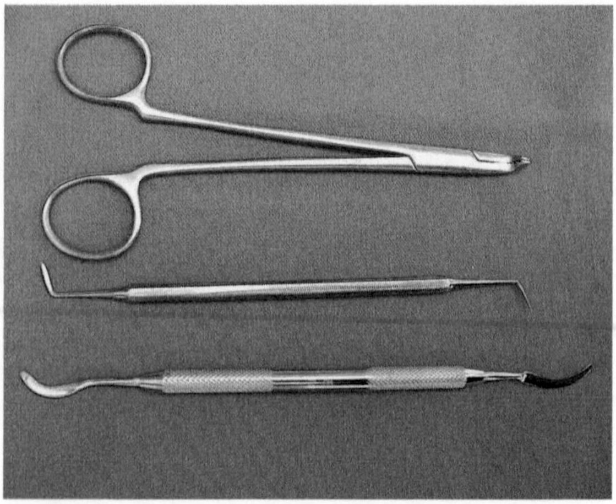

Fig. 12.17 Equipment 3 – extraction. From top to bottom: molar extraction forceps, Crossley molar luxator, Crossley incisor luxator.

Aradicular hypsodont incisor teeth

The most common indications for extraction of incisors are:

- Primary incisor overgrowth
- Periapical abscessation

Cheek teeth

Brachyodont

The pocket pets with brachyodont cheek teeth are spared the pathology associated with overgrowth of teeth. In our experience, the most common indication for tooth extraction is plaque-induced periodontal disease.

Aradicular hypsodont

The most common indication for extraction of cheek teeth is that they are affected by endodontic or periodontic disease resulting in periapical abscessation. Once a cheek tooth has been extracted, the patient will require long-term monitoring and regular trimming of the opposing teeth, as these will not wear down appropriately.

Summary

- Dental problems in lagomorphs and rodents are very common
- Most conditions are associated with incorrect husbandry and diet, and these issues must be addressed as part of the treatment
- These species are often presented late in the disease process, with consequent poorer prognosis
- Thorough intraoral examination requires general anaesthesia and radiography. Even under optimal conditions, some pathology may be missed
- Rabbits, guinea pigs and chinchillas with incisor overgrowth usually have a primary problem affecting the cheek teeth. Primary incisor overgrowth is considered rare except in young rabbits (less than one year of age)
- In guinea pigs, the problem is exacerbated by vitamin C deficiency. In chinchillas, it may be detected early by palpation of swellings on the ventral border of the mandible
- Rats, mice and hamsters with incisor overgrowth are not being given suitable food or substrate materials for gnawing
- Nail cutters are contraindicated for incisor shortening. As the problem is usually related to cheek teeth overgrowth, general anaesthesia is indicated
- Suitable equipment and instruments are needed for safe and effective tooth trimming in pocket pets

REFERENCES

Brown, S.A. & Rosenthal, K.L. (1997a) *Self Assessment Colour Review of Small Mammals*. London: Manson Publishing, pp. 77–78.

Crossley, D.A. (1995a) Clinical aspects of lagomorph dental anatomy: the rabbit (*Oryctolagus cuniculus*). *Journal of Veterinary Dentistry* **12**(4): 137–142.

Crossley, D.A. (1995b) Clinical aspects of rodent dental anatomy. *Journal of Veterinary Dentistry* **12**(4): 131–135.

Crossley, D.A. (2000) Rodent and rabbit radiology. In: DeForge, D.H. & Colmery, B.H. III (eds) *An Atlas of Veterinary Dental Radiology*. Ames, IA: Iowa State University Press, pp. 247–259.

Crossley, D.A. (2001) Dental disease in chinchillas in the UK. *Journal of Small Animal Practice* **42**(1): 12–19.

Crossley, D.A., Dubielzig, R.R. & Benson, K.G. (1997) Caries and odontoclastic resorptive lesions in a chinchilla (*Chinchilla laniger*). *Veterinary Record* **141**(27): 337–339.

Crossley, D.A., Jackson, A., Yates, J. & Boydell, I.P. (1998) Use of computed tomography to investigate cheek tooth abnormalities in chinchillas (*Chinchilla laniger*). *Journal of Small Animal Practice* **39**(8): 385–389.

Flecknell, P.A. (1991) Guinea pigs. In: Beynon, P.H. & Cooper, J.E. (eds) *Manual of Exotic Pets*. Cheltenham: BSAVA, pp. 52.

Harcourt-Brown, F.M. & Baker, S.J. (2001) Parathyroid hormone, haematological and biochemical parameters in relation to dental disease and husbandry in rabbits. *Journal of Small Animal Practice* **42**(3): 130–136.

Klaus, P. & Bennett, R.A. (1999) Management of abscesses of the head in rabbits. *Proceedings of the North American Veterinary Conference*, Orlando, USA.

Miles, A.E.W. & Crigson, C. (1990) *Colyer's Variations and Diseases of the Teeth of Animals*, revised edn. Cambridge: Cambridge University Press, pp. 567–569.

Redrobe, S. (1997) Surgical procedures and dental disorders. In: Flecknell, P. (ed) *Manual of Rabbit Medicine and Surgery*. Cheltenham: BSAVA, pp. 129–133.

Schaeffer, D.O. & Donnelly, T.M. (1997) Disease problems in guinea pigs and chinchillas. In: Hillyer, E.V. & Quesenberry, K.E. (eds) *Ferrets, Rabbits and Rodents: Clinical Medicine and Surgery*. Philadelphia: WB Saunders, pp. 260–281.

Wiggs, B. & Lobprise, H. (1995) Dental anatomy and physiology of pet rodents and lagomorphs. In: Crossley, D.A. & Penman, S. (eds) *Manual of Small Animal Dentistry*. Cheltenham: BSAVA, Ch. 7, pp. 68–73.

Williams, C.S.F. (1976) *Practical Guide to Laboratory Animals*. St Louis: Mosby.

Appendices

Appendix 1

Veterinary Nurses and the Veterinary Surgeons Act 1966

Introduction

1. Under the Veterinary Surgeons Act 1966 the general rule is that only a veterinary surgeon may practise veterinary surgery. There are, however, a number of exceptions to this rule, and two of them concern veterinary nurses. This note explains the law as it applies to them.

Definition of veterinary surgery

2. Veterinary surgery as defined in the Act 'means the art and science of veterinary surgery and medicine and, without prejudice to the generality of the foregoing, shall be taken to include:
   (a) the diagnosis of diseases in, and injuries to, animals including tests performed on animals for diagnostic purposes;
   (b) the giving of advice based upon such diagnosis;
   (c) the medical or surgical treatment of animals; and
   (d) the performance of surgical operations on animals.

Source: RCVS directory of registered veterinary nurses.

What can be done by people other than veterinary surgeons

3. Schedule 3 to the Act allows anyone to give first aid in an emergency for the purpose of saving life and relieving suffering. The owner of an animal, or a member of the owner's household or employee of the owner, may also give it minor medical treatment. There are a number of other exceptions to the general rule, mainly relating to farm animals, in addition to the exceptions which apply to veterinary nurses. These are explained below.

What can be done by veterinary nurses

4. Veterinary nurses, like anyone else, may give first aid and look after animals in ways which do not involve acts of veterinary surgery. In addition, veterinary nurses may do the things specified in paragraphs 6 and 7 of Schedule 3 to the Veterinary Surgeons Act 1966 as amended by the Veterinary Surgeons Act 1966 (Schedule 3 Amendment) Order 2002. The text of these paragraphs is set out in the annex below.

Listed veterinary nurses

5. Paragraph 6 applies to veterinary nurses whose names are entered on the list maintained by RCVS. They may administer

'any medical treatment or any minor surgery (not involving entry into a body cavity)' under veterinary direction.

6. The animal must be under the care of a veterinary surgeon and the treatment must be carried out at his or her direction. The veterinary surgeon must be the employer of the veterinary nurse or be acting on behalf of the nurse's employer.
7. The directing veterinary surgeon must be satisfied that the veterinary nurse is qualified to carry out the treatment or surgery. RCVS will advise from time to time on veterinary nursing qualifications which veterinary surgeons should recognise.
8. All listed veterinary nurses (VNs) are qualified to administer medical treatment or minor surgery (not involving entry into a body cavity), under veterinary direction, to all the species which are commonly kept as companion animals, including exotic species so kept. Unless they hold further qualifications they are not qualified to treat the equine species, wild animals or farm animals. Listed veterinary nurses who hold the RCVS Certificate in Equine Veterinary Nursing (EVNs) are qualified to administer medical treatment or minor surgery (not involving entry into a body cavity), under veterinary direction, to any of the equine species – horses, asses and zebras.
9. A veterinary nurse should only carry out a particular act of veterinary surgery if she or he is competent to do so and has the necessary experience to deal with any problems which may arise. Where appropriate, a veterinary surgeon should be available to respond to a request for help. A veterinary nurse may only carry out acts of veterinary surgery under the direction of a veterinary surgeon, who is accountable for what is done and should ensure that it is covered by professional indemnity insurance.

Student veterinary nurses

10. Paragraph 7 applies to student veterinary nurses. A student veterinary nurse is someone enrolled for the purpose of training as a veterinary nurse at an approved training and assessment centre (VNAC) or a veterinary practice approved by such a centre (TP). This does not include those who are undertaking the BVNA Pre-Veterinary Nursing Access Course.
11. A student veterinary nurse may administer 'any medical treatment or any minor surgery (not involving entry into a body cavity)' under veterinary direction.
12. The animal must be under the care of a veterinary surgeon and the treatment must be carried out at his or her direction. The veterinary surgeon must be the employer of the veterinary nurse or be acting on behalf of the nurse's employer.
13. The treatment or minor surgery must be carried out in the course of the student veterinary nurse's training. In the view of RCVS, such work should be undertaken only for the purpose of learning and consolidating new skills.
14. The treatment or surgery must be supervised by a veterinary surgeon or a listed veterinary nurse. In the case of surgery the supervision must be direct, continuous and personal.
15. In the view of RCVS, a veterinary surgeon or listed veterinary nurse can only be said to be supervising if they are present on the premises and able to respond to a request for assistance if needed. 'Direct, continuous and personal' supervision requires the supervisor to be present and giving the student nurse his or her undivided personal attention.

Medical treatment and minor surgery

16. The Act does not define 'any medical treatment or any minor surgery (not involving entry into a body cavity)'. Ultimately it would be for the courts to decide what these words mean.
17. The procedures which veterinary nurses are specifically trained to carry out include the following:
   - administer medication by mouth, topically, by the rectum, by inhalation or

by subcutaneous, intramuscular or intravenous injection;
- administer other treatments, including oral, intravenous and subcutaneous rehydration, other fluid therapy, catheterisation, cleaning and dressing of surgical wounds, treatment of abscesses and ulcers, application of external casts, holding and handling of viscera when assisting in operations and cutaneous suturing;
- prepare animals for anaesthesia and assist in the administration and termination of anaesthesia, including premedication, analgesia and intubation;
- collect samples of blood, urine, faeces, skin and hair; and
- take X-rays.

Guidance on anaesthesia

18. Particular care is needed over the administration of anaesthesia. A veterinary surgeon alone should:
    - assess the fitness of the animal to undergo anaesthesia;
    - select and plan a suitable anaesthetic regime;
    - select any premedication; and
    - administer anaesthetic if the induction dose is either incremental or to effect.
19. Provided the veterinary surgeon is physically present and immediately available for consultation, a listed veterinary nurse may:
    - administer selected sedative, analgesic or other agents before and after the operation;
    - administer non-incremental anaesthetic agents on the instruction of the directing veterinary surgeon;
    - monitor clinical signs and maintain an anaesthetic record; and
    - maintain anaesthesia by administering supplementary incremental doses of intravenous anaesthetic agents or adjusting the delivered concentration of anaesthetic agents, under the direct instruction of the supervising veterinary surgeon.

June 2002

Paragraphs 6 and 7 of Schedule 3 to the Veterinary Surgeons Act 1966, as amended by the Veterinary Surgeons Act 1966 (Schedule 3 Amendment) Order 2002, SI 2002/1479, with effect from 10 June 2002

6. Any medical treatment or any minor surgery (not involving entry into a body cavity) to any animal by a veterinary nurse if the following conditions are complied with, that is to say:
   (a) the animal is, for the time being, under the care of a registered veterinary surgeon or veterinary practitioner and the medical treatment or minor surgery is carried out by the veterinary nurse at his direction;
   (b) the registered veterinary surgeon or veterinary practitioner is the employer or is acting on behalf of the employer of the veterinary nurse; and
   (c) the registered veterinary surgeon or veterinary practitioner directing the medical treatment or minor surgery is satisfied that the veterinary nurse is qualified to carry out the treatment or surgery.

In this paragraph and in paragraph 7 below:

'veterinary nurse' means a nurse whose name is entered in the list of veterinary nurses maintained by the College.

7. Any medical treatment or any minor surgery (not involving entry into a body cavity) to any animal by a student veterinary nurse if the following conditions are complied with, that is to say:
   (a) the animal is, for the time being, under the care of a registered veterinary surgeon or veterinary practitioner and the medical treatment or minor surgery is carried out by the student veterinary nurse at his direction and in the course of the student veterinary nurse's training;

(b) the treatment or surgery is supervised by a registered veterinary surgeon, veterinary practitioner or veterinary nurse and, in the case of surgery, the supervision is direct, continuous and personal; and

(c) the registered veterinary surgeon or veterinary practitioner is the employer or is acting on behalf of the employer of the student veterinary nurse.

In this paragraph:

'student veterinary nurse' means a person enrolled under bye-laws made by the Council for the purpose of undergoing training as a veterinary nurse at an approved training and assessment centre or a veterinary practice approved by such a centre;

'approved training and assessment centre' means a centre approved by the Council for the purpose of training and assessing student veterinary nurses.

Appendix 2

Endodontics

Endodontics is the treatment of the pulp of the tooth (*endo-*: inside; *-dontic*: tooth).

There are three pulpal treatments, each of which has specific indications. They are:

1. Pulp capping
2. Partial pulpectomy with direct pulp capping
3. Root canal therapy.

Conventional root canal therapy is the most commonly indicated type of endodontic treatment. It involves total removal of pulp tissue, i.e. total pulpectomy, cleaning and filling of the root canal, followed by tooth restoration.

Root canal therapy is indicated when there is or may be irreversible pulp pathology (e.g. generalised pulpitis or pulp necrosis, often in combination with periapical involvement) in the mature permanent tooth. Immature permanent teeth are a special consideration and are dealt with separately.

The objectives of conventional root canal therapy are:

- To clean and disinfect the pulp chamber and root canals
- To fill the root canal(s) with a non-irritant, antibacterial material thus sealing the apex
- To close the access and exposure sites with a suitable restorative material

Many different methods are employed in the preparation and filling of root canals. In simple terms, root canal therapy involves removing the pulp, replacing it with an inert material and restoring the tooth. The inflamed or dead pulp is removed using special files. Once the pulp has been removed, the root canal is cleaned, both mechanically with files but also chemically with a disinfectant. The clean and disinfected root canal is then filled with inert material and the crown is restored with a suitable restorative material. The tooth is not restored to its original shape and size as the biting forces in the dog are much greater than those in humans and the restoration would be likely to fail if this was attempted.

The whole procedure is performed under general anaesthesia under strict radiographic control. It is time-consuming, as each step needs to be performed with meticulous detail to ensure successful outcome.

The outcome of conventional root canal therapy should be monitored radiographically for 6–12 months postoperatively. This will also require general anaesthesia. Evidence of disease around the tip of the root at this time indicates the need for further endodontic therapy or extraction of the tooth. Further endodontic therapy usually consists of redoing the root canal therapy, often in conjunction with surgical endodontics (usually removing the tip of the root and sealing the root canal from this direction as well).

Special considerations with immature teeth

A partial pulpectomy and direct pulp capping procedure is indicated for recent tooth crown fractures with pulp exposure in immature teeth. An immature tooth has a thin dentine wall and an open apex, allowing a good blood supply to the pulp. Treatment is aimed at maintaining a viable pulp, as this is needed for continued root development.

Necrotic immature teeth require endodontic treatment if they are to be retained. The procedure is an adaptation of conventional root canal therapy as already described for the mature permanent tooth. The necrotic pulp tissue is gently removed and the pulp chamber and root canal thoroughly cleaned. It is important to remove all the necrotic tissue, which usually extends slightly beyond the radiographically verifiable open apex. Sterile calcium hydroxide powder or paste is packed into the root canal, extending just beyond the apex. A degree of apexogenesis (normal root length and apex development) or apexification (treatment stimulated root closure) can be achieved if this procedure is performed. The exposure site is sealed with a restorative material. The tooth is monitored closely and the calcium hydroxide dressing is changed approximately every six months, as a fresh dressing is more effective in stimulating apexogenesis and apexification. When no further root development can be seen radiographically and if the apex is closed, a conventional root canal treatment should be performed. A conventional root canal treatment can only be carried out if the apex is closed. If the apex is still open and closure cannot be stimulated by repeated calcium hydroxide dressings, it may be possible to obtain an apical seal using a surgical approach and placing a root filling in a retrograde manner.

It must be noted that multiple general anaesthesia episodes are required and thus in most cases extraction of an immature tooth with a necrotic pulp is the best course of action. Salvage procedure as described above is really only indicated for the strategic permanent teeth that have undergone some degree of maturation.

It should be noted that immature teeth might well be present in the mature animal if trauma caused pulp necrosis during the developmental period. Treatment of such teeth is the same as for any immature permanent teeth, regardless of the actual age of the animal.

Glossary

Abrasion Wear of tooth surfaces that are not in contact with one another.

Alveolar bone Bone forming the sockets for the teeth.

Alveolar mucosa Oral mucosa that covers the alveolar processes.

Alveolar septum The dense bone separating alveoli of adjacent teeth.

Alveolus Socket within bone in which a tooth is normally located.

Ameloblast Cells that produce enamel (matrix).

Ameloblastoma Benign, but locally invasive neoplasm originating from odontogenic epithelium.

Anelodont Teeth which develop a true anatomical root structure and do not continuously grow throughout life.

Anisognathism Having upper and lower jaws of differing widths. Normal in most species.

Ankylosis (Greek for 'immobile') Fusion of bone and tooth substance along the root surface.

Anodontia The congenital absence of teeth.

Anterior Situated in front of. This term is commonly used to denote the incisor and canine teeth or the area toward the front of the mouth.

Anterior crossbite Reverse scissor occlusion of one, several or all of the incisors.

Apex Point or extremity of a conical object such as a tooth root.

Apexogenesis Normal root length and apex development.

Apical Direction toward the root tip or away from the incisal or occlusal surfaces.

Aradicular Without roots.

Aradicular hypsodont Dentition with long crowned teeth, without a true root structure, which are continually growing (e.g. lagomorphs, guinea pig, chinchilla). Elodont.

Attached gingiva Tightly attached gingiva extending from the free gingiva to the alveolar mucosa.

Attrition Wear of tooth surfaces that are in contact.

Avulsion Separation by traction. The dislocation of a tooth from its alveolus.

Bisecting angle Technique of taking radiographs to minimise linear distortion by aiming the beam perpendicular to the line that bisects the angle formed by the long axis of the tooth and the film.

Biting force The pressure exerted by teeth when engaged by the muscles of mastication.

Body of the mandible Horizontal portion of the mandible, excluding the alveolar process.

Brachycephalic Having a short skull, e.g. bulldogs, Pekinese.

Brachygnathism Having a short jaw.

Brachyodont Teeth that have a short crown : root ratio, with a true root.

Bruxism Abnormal grinding of the teeth.

Buccal Of, or towards, the cheek.

Buccal surface Surface of a posterior tooth positioned immediately adjacent to the cheek.

Bur A rotary instrument used for cutting and shaping teeth, bone, metal, etc.

Calculus Hard deposit which accumulates on the teeth. Mineralised plaque. Tartar.

Canines *See* cuspids.

Caries Progressive dissolution of tooth structure by bacterial acid and enzyme action. Common in humans, less common in dogs and not described in cats.

Carnassial teeth The largest shearing teeth in the upper and lower jaws (upper 4th premolar and lower 1st molar in dogs and cats).

Caudal Towards the tail. Away from the nose/head.

Cavity An abnormal hole or depression in the surface of a tooth, e.g. caries cavities and feline resorptive lesion cavities.

Cementoblasts Cells that form cementum.

Cemento-dentinal junction (CDJ) Junction where the cementum and dentine contact.

Cemento-enamel junction (CEJ) The line between anatomical root and crown where enamel ends, meeting the cementum covering the root. Term usually only used when referring to brachyodont teeth.

Cementum Bone-like connective tissue usually covering the surface of tooth roots and sometimes the crown; 65% mineral (calcium hydroxyapatite), 23% organic (mainly collagen), 12% water.

Cervical Of, or towards, the neck. Of that part of a tooth where root and crown meet.

Cheek teeth Term used to signify the premolar and/or molar teeth of herbivores as a functional unit.

Cheilitis Inflammation of the lips.

Chlorhexidine Chemical disinfectant often used for plaque control. Used as either the gluconate or acetate.

Cingulum The raised section or rudimentary cusp seen on the palatal or lingual surface of the crown of incisor teeth in humans and the dogs.

Clinical crown That portion of the tooth protruding above the gingiva.

Clinical root That portion of the tooth below the gingiva.

Congenital Present at birth.

Coronal Towards or pertaining to the crown of a tooth.

Curette Dental instrument used for removing plaque and calculus from the subgingival surface of tooth roots. Also used for root planing.

Cuspid (canine teeth, fang teeth) One of four pointed teeth situated one on each side of each jaw, immediately distal to the corner or lateral incisors.

Deciduous teeth Those teeth which are normally shed and replaced in diphyodont dentitions. Temporary, puppy, kitten, milk, baby or primary teeth.

Dental abrasion Wear from the friction of an externally applied force, such as brushing.

Dental attrition Wear or loss of tooth substance due to normal masticatory forces, i.e. teeth that are in contact.

Dental luxator Instrument with a wider, but more delicate blade than an elevator that is used in the periodontal space to sever the periodontal ligament attachment.

Dentine (dentin) Hard connective tissue forming main bulk of most teeth; 70% mineral (calcium hydroxyapatite), 18% organic (mainly collagen), 12% water.

Dentino-enamel junction (DEJ) Juncture within the crown of the tooth where the dentinal and enamel walls meet.

Dentition Name used to signify the characteristics, arrangement and function of teeth, e.g. carnivorous, herbivorous and omnivorous dentition.

Developer Solution to make the latent image on an exposed X-ray film visible.

Diastema A natural gap or space between teeth in the same jaw. Examples include the space between the incisors and cheek teeth in lagomorphs and rodents; and the space between maxillary incisors and canine teeth in carnivores.

Diphyodont Dentition where one set of teeth (the deciduous dentition) is shed, being replaced by a second set (the permanent dentition).

Disclosing agents Organic dyes capable of indicating the presence of plaque.

Disinfectants Agents which remove or kill microorganisms.

Distal Farthest away from. Away from the median point of the dental arch. The actual direction varies along the dental arch.

Distal surface Surface of a tooth facing away from the median line following the curve of the dental arch.

Dolichocephalic Having a long skull, as seen in rough collies and Dobermans.

Dysplasia Abnormal development, for example enamel dysplasia.

Elodont Teeth which grow throughout life. Aradicular hypsodont teeth.

Enamel Very hard outer layer of tooth crown in humans and carnivores; 96% mineral (calcium hydroxyapatite), 2% protein (enamelin), 2% water.

Enamel hypoplasia Condition in which the enamel is abnormal.

Enamel organ Ectodermal epithelial structure that leads to the formation of tooth enamel.

Endodontic Of or pertaining to the tissue within a tooth, i.e. the pulp/dentine unit.

Enzymatic toothpaste Dentifrice containing enzymes which enhance the natural salivary plaque control mechanisms.

Epiglottis Mucosal-covered cartilage that helps cover the laryngeal opening.

Epithelial attachment Cells that attach the gingiva to the tooth.

Epulis Clinical descriptive term for mass on gingiva.

Eruption Movement of a tooth as it emerges through surrounding tissue so that the clinical crown gradually appears longer.

Exfoliation Shedding or loss of a primary tooth.

External resorption Destruction of dental hard tissues which starts on the external root surfaces and progresses within the tooth.

Extract To pull out or remove.

Facial The outward facing, labial and buccal, surfaces of the teeth.

Facial nerve Cranial nerve VII.

Fauces Region lateral to the palato-glossal folds bilaterally.

Fibrosarcoma Malignant neoplasm. Common in dogs.

Fixer solutions Used to preserve and enhance the latent image on the radiographic film.

Fossa A shallow depression, e.g. the depression between the cingulum and incisal edge of certain incisor teeth.

Frenulum Fold of alveolar mucosa forming a noticeable ridge of attachment, e.g. between the lips and gums and below the tongue and floor of the mouth.

Fulcrum Centre of rotation of the tooth, usually occurring approximately at the junction of the middle and apical thirds of the root.

Functional occlusion Active tooth contacts during mastication and swallowing; also called dynamic occlusion.

Furcation Forking or branching point. Bifurcation or trifurcation: the area where the roots of multirooted teeth meet.

Fusion The joining of two or more teeth each retaining its own structure.

Gemination The partial splitting of a tooth giving the appearance of a double crown whilst having a single root structure.

Gingiva Connective tissue cuff around each tooth. Gum.

Gingival Of or pertaining to the gingiva.

Gingival crest Most occlusal or incisal extent of gingiva.

Gingival fibres Connective tissue fibres in the gingiva.

Gingival fluid Tissue fluid which exudes through the sulcular epithelium.

Gingival hyperplasia Proliferation of the attached gingiva.

Gingival margin Crest of gingiva around the tooth.

Gingival papilla Gingival tissue in the interproximal space between two adjacent teeth.

Gingival pocket Abnormal, pathological space between the tooth root and gingiva.

Gingival sulcus Gap or potential space situated between the free gingiva and the tooth surface.

Gingivectomy Excision of excessive gingival tissues to create a new gingival margin.

Gingivitis Inflammation of the gingiva.

Gnathic Of the jaw. In general use refers to the mandible.

Gum In common usage – gingiva.

Halitosis Unpleasant breath odour.

Hard palate Bony vault of the oral cavity proper covered with soft tissue.

Hereditary Term describing traits received from past ancestors that produce specific characteristics.

Heterodont Dentition comprising teeth of different shapes and function.

High speed Used to describe air driven turbine mechanisms capable of rotation at over 100 000 revolutions per minute (rpm). Typical high speed handpieces rotate burs at around 200 000 rpm.

Homodont The feature of having teeth that are all of the same general shape or type, although size may vary, as in fish, reptiles and sharks.

Hypodontia Condition in which some teeth are missing.

Hypoplastic enamel Thin enamel, commonly seen in conjunction with enamel hypocalcification.

Hypsodont Dentition comprising long crowned teeth, radicular or aradicular.

Impacted tooth A tooth which cannot erupt, or complete its eruption, due to contact with an obstruction such as another tooth.

Incisal Coronal portion or direction in incisors.

Incisal bone The premaxilla, rostral most area of upper jaw that accommodates the maxillary incisors.

Incisors Centre teeth in either arch that are essential for cutting.

Infrabony pocket Periodontal pocket that has its base apical to the alveolar crest; also known as sub-alveolar pocket.

Interdental Situated between adjacent teeth.

Interdental papillae Projection of gingiva between the teeth.

Interdental septum Bone between the roots of adjacent teeth.

Internal resorption Destruction of dental hard tissues which starts on the pulpal surface and extends towards the external aspects of the tooth.

Interproximal Between adjoining surfaces of adjacent teeth.

Interproximal space Space between adjoining teeth.

Interradicular fibres Alveolodental periodontal ligament fibres in multirooted teeth that go from the interradicular crestal bone to cementum.

Intraradicular septum Bone between the roots of multirooted teeth.

Intrusion Movement of the tooth further into the alveolus.

Irreversible pulpitis Inflammation of the pulp that cannot be resolved, leading to the death of the vital pulp.

Junctional epithelium Epithelium that acts to hold mucosa in the base of the gingival sulcus to the tooth.

Labial Of, towards, or pertaining to the lips.

Labial surface Surface of an anterior tooth positioned immediately adjacent to the lip.

Lamina dura Radiographic term denoting the cribriform plate, bundle bone, and the dense alveolar bone surrounding a root.

Level bites When the incisor teeth meet edge on edge or the premolars or molars occlude cusp to cusp.

Lingual Of, towards, or pertaining to the tongue.

Lingual surface Surface of a tooth immediately adjacent to the tongue.

Low speed Dental engines or handpieces capable of providing rotation up to 30 000 revolutions per minute.

Luxation Dislocation of a joint. Partial or complete separation of a tooth from its alveolus.

Macrodontia Having larger teeth than normal.

Malocclusion Abnormal tooth positioning.

Mandible Lower jaw.

Mandibular Pertaining to the lower jaw.

Mandibular symphysis Point at which the mandibular processes fuse, forming the mandible.

Mastication Act of chewing or grinding.

Maxillae Paired main bones of the upper jaw.

Maxillary Pertaining to the upper arch.

Medial/Median Towards/at the midline of the body.

Mental foramen Foramen on the lateral side of the mandible, below the premolars.

Mesial Towards the point of the dental arch situated in the median plane.

Mesial surface Surface of a tooth facing toward the median line, following the curve of the dental arch.

Mesocephaly Condition marked by a balanced facial profile, somewhere between dolichocephalic and brachycephalic, as in beagles and German shepherds.

Microdontia Having smaller teeth than normal.

Milk teeth Those teeth which are normally shed and replaced in diphyodont dentitions. Primary, temporary, deciduous, puppy, kitten or baby teeth

Mixed dentition The feature of having primary and permanent teeth in the dental arches at the same time.

Molars Teeth with occlusal surface that can be used to grind food or break it down into smaller pieces.

Monophydont Having one set of teeth, i.e. permanent, only.

Mucogingival junction The line between attached gingiva and oral mucosa.

Occluding Contacting opposing teeth.

Occlusal Of or pertaining to the surface of a tooth which meets a tooth in the opposite jaw, e.g. the occlusal surfaces of molar teeth.

Occlusal plane The angles of the upper and lower jaws in relation to each other.

Occlusal surface Surface of a premolar or molar within the marginal ridges that contacts the corresponding surfaces of antagonists during closure of the posterior teeth.

Occlusal trauma Injury caused by malocclusion.

Occlusion Coming together. The relationship of upper and lower teeth.

Odontoblasts Cells that form dentine.

Oligodontia Having fewer teeth than normal.

Oral epithelium Lining membrane of the oral cavity consisting of stratified squamous epithelium.

Oral mucosa Stratified squamous epithelium running from the margins of the lips to the area of the tonsils and lining the oral cavity; also known as oral mucous membrane.

Orthodontics Study and treatment relating to restoration of normal tooth position and jaw relationships.

Osteoblasts Cells that form bone.

Osteoclasts Multinucleated cells responsible for destroying bone, as well as cementum and dentine.

Palatal Pertaining to the palate or roof of the mouth.

Palatal surface Lingual (medial) surface of maxillary teeth.

Palate Roof of the mouth.

Peg teeth The small 2nd maxillary incisors, located behind the large 1st maxillary incisors, in lagomorphs.

Pellicle Amorphous coating of salivary proteins and glycoproteins attached to exposed tooth surfaces in the mouth.

Periapical Around the tip of a tooth root.

Periodontal Around or surrounding teeth and their roots. Of, or pertaining to, the periodontium.

Periodontal disease Plaque induced inflammation of periodontium. Includes gingivitis and periodontitis.

Periodontal membrane or ligament Connecting tissue connecting the tooth to the alveolar bone.

Periodontitis Plaque induced inflammation of the periodontal tissues resulting in destruction of probing depth and alveolar bone.

Periodontium Periodontal tissues. Tissues adjacent to, surrounding and supporting the tooth and its roots. Alveolar bone, periodontal ligament, cementum and gingiva.

Permanent teeth Final or lasting set of teeth that are typically of a very durable and lasting nature (opposite of deciduous).

Physiological mobility Degree of tooth movement that can be considered normal.

Plaque Biofilm composed of aggregates of bacteria and their by-products, salivary components, oral debris and occasional epithelial and inflammatory cells.

Posterior Situated toward the back, such as premolars and molars.

Posterior crossbite Term used to describe an abnormal relationship of the carnassial teeth, where the normal buccolingual relationship is reversed.

Pre-eruptive stage Period of time when the crown of the tooth is developing, before tooth erupts into oral cavity.

Premaxilla Bony area of the upper jaw that includes the alveolar ridge for the incisors and the area immediately behind it in primates.

Premolars Teeth designed to help hold and carry, like cuspids, and break food down into smaller pieces, like molars; also known as bicuspids.

Primary teeth The first tooth to appear in each position in the mouth. In diphyodont animals these include the deciduous teeth *plus* those permanent teeth without deciduous precursors.

Prognathism Having a longer or protruding jaw, e.g. relative mandibular prognathism.

Proximal Close to or towards the centre or midline.

Proximal surface Surface of a tooth facing toward an adjoining tooth in the same arch (e.g. both mesial and distal surfaces are proximal surfaces).

Pseudopockets False gingival pockets in which gingival height is increased due to hyperplasia, resulting in deeper 'pocket' readings but without attachment loss.

Ptyalism Excessive salivation, usually with excess drooling from mouth (slobbers).

Pulp Soft tissue within a tooth composed of odontoblasts, nerves, blood vessels, lymphatics and connective tissue.

Pulp canal Root canal. The space within a tooth root running from the apex to the pulp chamber.

Pulp cavity The pulp canal and chamber.

Pulp chamber The space within a tooth crown occupied by pulp tissue.

Pulpal exposure Unnatural opening of the pulp chamber by pathological or mechanical means.

Pulpal necrosis Partial or total pulpal death.

Pulpectomy Extirpation of the entire pulp.

Pulpitis Inflammation of pulp tissue – may be caused by thermal, chemical, infective or traumatic insults.

Pulpectomy Surgical removal of the pulp.

Radicular Of or pertaining to the (tooth) root.

Radicular hypsodont Tooth with long anatomical crown and comparatively short root. The tooth grows for most of the animal's life, but late in life, the root apex closes and the tooth growth ceases, e.g. cows, horses.

Recession Migration of the gingival crest in an apical direction, away from the crown of the tooth.

Reparative dentine Dentine deposited as a result of injury or irritation to the pulp. Tertiary dentine.

Resorption Physiological removal of tissues or body products, as of the roots of deciduous teeth or of some alveolar process after the loss of the permanent teeth.

Restorative dentistry The study of, or treatment involving, the replacement of lost or missing tooth structure.

Root That part of the tooth normally remaining in the alveolus.

Root bifurcation The point at which a root trunk divides into two separate branches.

Root exposure Uncovering or exposing of root surfaces due to periodontal tissue loss.

Root planing Procedure for smoothing the cementum of the root of a tooth.

Root trifurcation The point at which a root trunk divides into three separate branches.

Rostral Towards the nose. Away from the tail.

Rugae Small ridges of tissue extending laterally across the anterior of the hard palate.

Scaler Dental instrument used for the removal of plaque and calculus from the crowns of teeth. Hand scaler, ultrasonic scaler, sonic scaler.

Scissor bite Normal relationship of the maxillary incisors overlapping the mandibular incisors whose incisal edges rest on or near the cingulum on the lingual surfaces on the maxillary incisors.

Secondary dentine Physiological deposition of dentine throughout life.

Secondary dentition Permanent dentition.

Slobbers Ptyalism causing fur to be wet and matted around the mouth, jaw and ventral neck, particularly in chinchillas.

Soft palate Unsupported soft tissue that extends back from the hard palate free of the support of the palatine bone.

Stomatitis Inflammation of the soft tissues of the oral cavity or mouth.

Subgingival curettage Removal of diseased soft tissue within a periodontal pocket.

Subluxation Incomplete dislocation of a joint, such as the temporomandibular joint or a tooth.

Supernumerary teeth Extra teeth, above the normal number. Often seen in the incisor region in brachycephalic dogs and the premolar region of dolicocephalic dogs.

Tartar *See* calculus.

Temporary teeth Deciduous teeth.

Temporomandibular joint (TMJ) Joint composed of the condylar process of the vertical ramus of the mandible and the mandibular fossa of the temporal bone of the skull.

Tertiary dentine Dentine deposited as a result of injury or irritation to the pulp. Reparative dentine.

Toothbrushing Mechanical means of removing dental plaque.

Version Angulation. Bucco-, linguo-, labio-, palato-version; angulation of a tooth or teeth with the crown deviated towards the cheek, tongue, lip, palate.

Vestibule That part of the mouth between the teeth and the lips/cheek.

Wet dewlap Moist dermatitis on the ventral neck of rabbits from ptyalism due to malocclusion, stomatitis or other oral inflammation. Slobbers.

Xerostomia Dry mouth, due to lack of salivary secretion.

Index

R

S

Printed and bound by CPI Group (UK) Ltd, Croydon, CR0 4YY
03/10/2024
01040349-0013